# Nature Power

*AuthorHouse™ UK Ltd.*
*1663 Liberty Drive*
*Bloomington, IN 47403 USA*
*www.authorhouse.co.uk*
*Phone: 0800.197.4150*

*Published by AuthorHouse    09/30/2013*

*ISBN: 978-1-4918-7834-7 (sc)*
*ISBN: 978-1-4918-7851-4 (e)*

*Cover Photo: by Pax Herbal Center, Nigeria*

# Nature Power

## Natural Medicine in Tropical Africa

yr. 2018

M. E. Aisabokhae

*Anselm Adodo, OSB*

authorHOUSE®

# DEDICATION

*To Life*

# CONTENTS

- Knowledge without local substance
- Functional knowledge
- Danger of fragmented knowledge
- A new world

- Re-educating our children about herbal medicine
- Herbalism
- Our cultural traditions are not inferior
- The problem of nomenclature
- Finding a balance
- What is the goal of medicine?
- Why do we fall sick?
- What is a drug?
- What is a medicine?
- Energy is ability
- What is thermodynamics?
- Some criticisms of herbal medicines
- Uses of herbs
- Criticism revisited
- Herbal medicine in Britain
- Herbal medicine in the United States of America
- What is cure?
- The Price of 'cure'
- What is alternative medicine?
- What is complementary medicine?
- What is 'cam'?
- Evidence–based medicine
- Do herbs have side-effects?

- When to harvest herbs
- How to harvest herbs
- How to dry herbs
- How to take herbs

- Psalm of thank you
- Health benefits of bitter leaf
- The Wonders of Pawpaw
- The Life Giving Properties of Water
- The Medicinal Value of Coconut
- Aloe Vera: The Wonder Plant
- Herbal Cure for Diabetes
- Arthritis is Curable with Herbs
- Lemon - The Tree of Life
- Mistletoe: Nature's Potent Cure All
- The Healing Powers of Garlic
- Ginger: The Aromatic Herb
- Urine as Medicine
- The Many uses of Plantain
- Healing with Carrot
- The Healing Properties of Avocado Pear

- The Healing Potency of Sound
- Medicine for Death
- Vibration Medicine
- Spiritual Radiotherapy: An Approach to Cancer Treatment

- What is Radiation?
- What is Radiotherapy?
- What is Cancer?
- Symptoms of Cancer
- Common Cancers in Nigeria
- What causes Cancer?
- The Material Order
- The mental/ Spiritual Order
- The Cosmic Order
- Cancer: The Water Connection

- Let Me Be
- Getting used to Colours

- Typhoid Fever
- Malaria Fever
- Peptic Ulcer
- Hepatitis
- Anemia
- Chest and Waist Pain
- Kidney Problem
- Internal Heat
- Glaucoma
- Dysentery
- Bronchitis
- Indigestion

- Ulcer (External)
- Scabies
- Lumbago
- Stroke
- Measles
- Insomnia
- Jaundice
- Migraine
- Epilepsy
- Pile
- Depression
- Pneumonia
- Tuberculosis
- Hypertension

- Psalm 8
- The Glory of Womanhood
- The Problem of Infertility
- The Pain of Impotence
- Coping with Menopause

- The Dance of Life
- The River of Life

# PREFACE

Before the colonial age, medicine across the tropics was almost entirely confined to traditional remedies and practices tailored to local cultures and natural resources. Then the arrival of missionaries and colonialists in Asia, Africa and America brought modern scientific techniques and medicines that were used to serve the colonial imperative of promoting Christianity, commerce and "civilisation".

The introduction of modern medicine has certainly been successful on one level. The colonial powers were much more adept at controlling epidemics, deploying mass vaccination programmes against smallpox, for example, and removing tumours and cataracts. However, colonial-era medicine has left another legacy—the marginalisation and downgrading of traditional medicine. Colonial powers promoted their values over traditional practices, establishing modern medicine as officially superior. In many African countries for example, herbalists were not forbidden to practice but they were largely considered inferior or ignored.

This marginalisation of traditional medical practices was later reinforced through organised healthcare systems and hospitals built on developed countries' models, which have continued to dominate the healthcare systems of most nations. Fortunately, in the race to meet the Millennium Development Goals, combat increasing drug resistance and tackle new diseases, traditional medicine is making a comeback! Governments, drug companies, researchers and international aid organisations increasingly recognise the value of traditional medicine and its practitioners.

When *Nature Power* was first published 13 years ago, the practice of herbal medicine in Nigeria and in most parts of Africa was identified with witchcraft, sorcery, ritualism and all sorts of fetish practices. Because herbal medicine was associated with paganism, many African Christians secretly patronize traditional healers, and the educated elite and religious figures did not want to be associated in any way with traditional African Medicine. *Nature Power*, like a lonely voice in a wilderness, was written to correct the misconception that African Herbal medicine is synonymous with paganism, ritualism and fetishism.

Since its publication, *Nature Power* has been reprinted and revised more than eight times. It has contributed immensely in changing the attitudes of both the Government and Christians towards the practice of herbal medicine. *Nature Power* has also helped to show that health is more than an absence of disease. Health is wholeness of mind, soul and body. Much of the information in this book are age-old secrets, which herbalists keep close to their chests. I have made them available here so that humanity may profit from them.

It is said that knowledge is power. True enough. But knowledge is power only when it is relevant and makes a difference in the lives of people. *Nature Power* has indeed made a big difference in the lives of the people!

When God made men and women, he gave them all they needed to be happy, to be whole, and to be healthy. He gave water, air, the earth and us sunshine. Out of greed and selfishness, we began to exploit the earth, abuse it, destroy it, and treat it with disrespect. The result is crisis: economic crisis, mental crisis, social crisis, political crisis and climatic crisis. The world is in crisis because it is populated by over 6 billion greedy individuals: you and I.

We who are adults know that we have lost our childhood innocence, and we know that somehow, our happiness depends on regaining it. Somehow, we know that we have lost touch with nature, and somewhere deep in our hearts we know that we need to get in touch with nature. We human beings are the youngest occupants of this planet. Before we came, the plants were here; before we came, the animals were here; before we came, the oceans, the forests, and the mountains were here. To survive, we must learn from her. In addition, to learn from her, we must respect her.

Nature Power is inviting the world to come down to the earth to regain our health. We are people of the earth. The earth is the primary source of our creativity, intelligence and human-ness. Before we set out to calculate, to create, to invent, to fabricate, the earth already was. Science does not and cannot create. Science only tries to explain nature, to interpret it, manage it, mimic it, control it, exploit it and do all kinds of things with it. People go to school to learn about nature, to understand it, to explain it. They acquire degrees, become experts, professionals and professors in various fields of human Knowledge: medicine, physics, chemistry, pharmacy, botany, biology, astronomy, geography, psychology, engineering, architecture, etc. Call it what you wish, describe it as you like, explain it as you want, mystify it as you please, it still boils down to the same thing: **NATURE.**

We must remain close to the earth, so that we do not lose contact with our roots, our origin. Today, faced with globalization, high-technology and a fast-paced modern lifestyle, we are often tempted to forget our link with the earth, and therefore become DIS-EASED. One distinctive feature of nature is that it is generous; it is an open book, open for everyone to read and understand. In addition, the more we learn about nature, the more our knowledge grows, and the wiser we become. Moreover, the wiser we become, the more our need to know more increases.

In the past, we used to hear about physicians who provide health *care* to the sick. Physicians who genuinely *care* for the sick. Today, it seems what we have are more of health specialists or professionals, who help us fix our bodies when broken down so that we can keep on moving. Yes, they may have cured us, but do they really *care*? Is health care in the modern world becoming more of a business venture rather than a *care* profession? And what about the botanist and taxonomist who, while gaining a technical knowledge of trees and plants, have lost knowledge of the forest? Or the astronaut who, while becoming an expert in the study of the moon and the stars, has lost knowledge of the sky? Before our very eyes, we observe experts and professionals taking over our lives, controlling it, and forming a powerful clique with a claim to a monopoly of knowledge, and restricting our access to the open book, which is nature.

I invite all men and women of goodwill to show some concern about the quality of advice given to government by our so-called experts and ask some vital questions. Is government getting the right advice concerning health care and how to improve it? Has importation of sophisticated machines into our hospitals in Africa translated into more efficient health care and treatment?

Does bigger spending really translate into better health services? In villages where there are no roads, no electricity, no hospitals, what form of health care should government put in place? Since the current health system in operation in Nigeria and many African countries has not fully met the health needs of the people, what alternative do we have? Is government ready and willing to explore and embrace the alternative? Do we honestly believe that the health care model of the developed and industrialised countries of Europe and America is suitable to, or is practicable in Africa?

Our health, our life, our future, depends on the quality of the earth: soil, water, sunshine, forests and air. The rich, the poor, the sick, the healthy, black people, white people, we all breathe the same air. There is no separate air for different categories of people. At the end of the day, what we put into the earth will come back to us, either to purify us or poison us. The air we breathe is the same air inhaled by Jesus Christ, by the Blessed Virgin Mary, by Mohammed, and by the great scientists, philosophers and saints of the past. Their utterances, thoughts and breath are still present in the air molecules in which we are immersed. So long as we all breathe the same air, and live on the same planet earth, we will all remain bonded together, both the living and the dead. Viewed from this perspective, one can now see how scientific our African ancestors were when they asserted that only a thin line separates the spiritual from the physical, spirit from matter, life from death. The wisdom of the ancients is there in the molecules of the air around us, waiting to be tapped when we are open enough to perceive it.

The idea of the stranger, the unknown, is an illusion. We are all linked together in a symbiotic cosmos. What affects one, affects all. Nobody is destined to be poor, or to be sick. We cannot sit down and watch politicians dictate the tempo of our lives and tell us what they want us to hear. People all over the world are challenging capitalism itself, a system that is based on intense greed, selfishness and competition. Privileged elite numbering a few thousands possess and have acquired over 80% of world's wealth and leave the remaining 5.6 billion people to scramble for the remaining 20%.

Millions of men and women from all parts of the world are coming together to remind us that it is our human greed and selfishness, rather than nuclear bombs, that constitute the greatest threat to human survival, to human health and to human peace. Humanity is sick and needs to be administered the medicine of justice, fairness, concern for others and respect for our symbiotic cosmos.

Over the past few years, there have been intense calls from readers to make the *Nature Power* available to the global reading public, as its message is as relevant today as it was 13 years ago. This new, expanded edition of *Nature power* is in response to this request. I hope it will be as profitable for you as it has been for millions of readers over the past decade.

# TERMINOLOGY

| Term | Meaning |
|------|---------|
| Bottle | Bear bottle (approximately 600ml) |
| Glass | 2.50ml(The common handless used for drinking) |
| Tablespoon | 10-15ml (tablespoon Dessertspoon are used synonymously) |
| Handfuls | The amount of fresh or dry leaves or roots that you can hold in your fist. |
| Twice Daily | In the morning and in the evening |
| 1 Liter | 1½ Beer Bottle (Approximately 1000ml) |

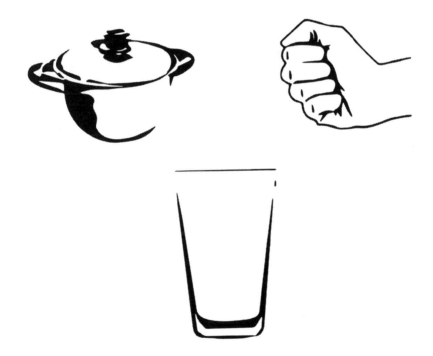

# CHAPTER ONE

# THE GOSPEL OF NATURAL MEDICINE

## *Song of Creation*

*In the beginning God created heaven and earth.*
*Now the earth was a formless void.*
*There was darkness over the deep,*
*And the spirit of God was hovering over the waters*

*God said: "Let there be light,"*
*And there was light.*

*God saw that the light was good*
*And He separated the light from the darkness.*
*God said: "Let there be a vault"*
*To separate the waters in two.*
*The vault became the heavens,*
*And God saw that it was good.*

*God said: "Let the earth produce vegetation,"*
*And there came cocoyam and banana,*
*Pawpaw, Orange and Guava,*
*And God saw that it was good.*

*God said: "Let living creatures come forth,"*
*And suddenly snakes, dogs and rabbits appeared,*
*Sheep, goats, lions and monkeys moved about,*
*And God saw that it was good.*

*God said: "Let us make man and woman."*
*God created them in God's own image,*
*And when God saw the beauty of God's creation*
*God danced for joy.*

## Waking Up

*Wake up, sleeper, Rise from the dead, and*
*Christ will shine on you (Eph. 4:14)*

Are you asleep? Why not wake up today? The cock crows, the snake hisses, the Lion roars, the birds sing. Singing the song of liberation, the song of freedom. Can you hear it? Wake up o sleeper and come back to your senses. This book is an invitation, a clarion call from a human being like you, to wake up and become the person you are meant to be. This is a message of hope from your fellow human being in search of knowledge, happiness, wholeness and peace. From one who believes in life and the sacredness of the Cosmos and everything in it. I am your fellow seeker after truth. I am not one who has more knowledge than you have, or more superior in the things of the spirit. I am only a storyteller. Is anybody ready to listen? I am only a singer, but is anybody willing to sing? I am a drummer, but is anyone ready to dance?

## Telling the Story

Once upon a time, there was a man who had a wife and ten children. He was a happy man. Every year, he would take his wife and children far away into the forest. On arriving there he would sit them down together, teach them how to beat the drum, how to dance the dance, how to sing the song and finally, how to tell the story. They would go back home happy, because the story linked them to their beginning. Shortly after, the man died, his children came together and said, "We do not know the way to the forest, so let us stay at home and beat the drum, dance the dance, sing the song and tell the story." So they did, and they were happy. Shortly after, the children died. Their children came together and said, "We do not know the way to the forest, neither do we know how to beat the drum. Let us stay at home and dance the dance, sing the song and tell the story". So they did, and they were fulfilled, for they found meaning in the story. Soon, the children's children also died, and the generation after them came together and said, "We do not know the way to the forest, neither can we beat the drum nor dance the dance. Let us stay at home and sing the song and tell the story." So they did, and they were healed, for the story made them feel at one with the cosmos. Soon, this generation died, and those after them came together and said, "We are the most unfortunate of all. We do not know the way to the forest, neither can we beat the drum, nor dance, nor sing. All we have left is the story. Let us then tell the story, so that we can be made whole. So they did, and were transformed."

We, the people of today . . . we have lost everything! All we have left is the story. The day we lose the story, is the day it is all over for us. We need prophets, visionaries and mystics to keep reminding us. To keep retelling the story. To keep on singing the song. To keep on dancing the dance. Modern men and women need to keep retelling their story. So that they may live.

### Who Are You?

So tell me, mortal man, who are you? You are nothing. Do you know that? You are nothing. A mere shadow passing by. Look at your life. What does it consist of? You are born. You grow up. You go to school. You become a lawyer, or a doctor, or a politician. You marry a wife (or two). You buy a car. You build a house. You fall sick and spend your hard-earned money in getting yourself cured. Yet, you die anyway, and you are buried. Is that not all? Tell me, o mortal human, who are you?

How proud we human beings are! We make ourselves the center of the universe. We separate ourselves from the universe, thinking that everything is under our control. We exploit the cosmos and treat it as we like, thinking that we really understand the mysteries of the world. Just because we manufacture airplanes and cars, because we make rockets that fly in the sky, because we manufacture atomic and chemical weapons (which can destroy our children and us), we think we are God! Whether we accept it or not, this is the truth . . . you are nothing.

*Sheer futility, Qoheleth says. Sheer*
*Futility: Everything is futile! What*
*Profit can we show for all our toil,*
*toiling under the sun? A generation*

*goes, a generation comes, yet the
earth stands firm forever . . . I thought
to myself, "very well, I will try
pleasure and see what enjoyment has
to offer." And this was futile too . . . I
resolved to embrace folly, to discover
the best way for people to spend their
days under the sun. I worked on a
grand scale: built myself palaces,
planted vineyards, made myself
gardens and orchards, I amassed
silver and gold, the treasures of kings
and provinces; acquired singers, men
and women, and every human luxury,
chest upon chest of it . . . I then
reflected on all that my hands had
achieved and all the effort I had put
into its achieving. What futility it all
was what chasing after the wind!
[Ecclesiastes. Chapter 1, verses1-4;
Chapter 2, verses1& 4; Chapter 8,
verse 11]*

### You Are a Voice

You are a voice of God. You are a language of God. God uttered you into existence. You are a phrase or a sentence in the cosmic story told by the grand Story Teller-God. You are not an accident. You are a part of the story of the cosmos. Just as the absence of an important phrase or sentence can spoil a story; the story of the universe is not complete without you. Do you know that? Your happiness lies in being what you are. Unhappiness lies in becoming what you are not. You are a part of the cosmos, but you are not the cosmos. You are an essential note in the Sacred Music, which is the cosmos, for a missing note is enough to spoil the music.

### You Are Somebody

Without Christ you are nothing. Without Christ all is futile. No peace, no happiness. You would only feel emptiness, pain and sorrow. But with Christ, life is worth living. In Christ, you are somebody. You are a saint. Do you now understand? Christ is the meaning of your life. Christ is the basis of your existence. Christ is the primordial voice with which you were uttered. Christ is the light that lightens the darkness in the world.

> *The Word was the real light*
> *That gives light to everyone*
> *He was coming into the world.*
> *He was in the world*
> *That had come into being through Him*
> *And the world did not recognized Him (Jn. 1:8-9)*

In Christ, God is made manifest. All that you need to know about God has been revealed in Christ, who is the way to God. It is only in Christ that you can discover who you are. When you pray, do not say, "Reveal Yourself to me O God". Rather say, "Reveal me to myself, O God". Do not say, "When I get to heaven, I will see God face to face." Instead, say, "When I see God face to face, I am in heaven."

My adventure into the world of natural therapy, which involves herbal medicine, is a mission. This is a mission to set our people free from ignorance, to open the eyes of the blind in order to see the hands of oppression, injustice and exploitation and to fight against them. Natural medicine is not just about the physical wellbeing of the person. It is rather, a call to a total liberation of the person; body, mind and soul. It is a call to resist the systematic exploitation of the poor by the rich, to care for the Cosmos, and protect it against pollution and destruction. May this little work be a contribution towards making this world a better place and restoring the dignity of creation.

## A New Beginning

In the beginning was life. Life spoke and there was life. Life brought life into being. The universe, the sky, the oceans, the hills, the mountains, the animals, the spirits and human beings came into being. Because life spoke. Life made life to be. Life expresses itself in life. Life manifests and reveals itself in various ways and with different intensities. Life manifests itself in the mountains, the sky, plants and animals. Creation is an echo of life.

Plants and animals are not unaware of the existence of each other. There is constant communication and interaction between human beings and the spirit. Every creation is linked with every other creature. For life cannot be separated from life.

Human beings have more life than plants and animals because they have minds and consciousness of their own. The forest, river, plants and animals interact in a non-conscious or unreflective way. But human beings have awareness and are conscious of their consciousness. Human beings have the capacity to become gods.

## The African Universe

The African Universe is a world of relationships, of interaction between the living and the dead, between the natural and supernatural. A community is not just a place where human beings dwell. The African community comprises of plants, animals, human beings, the spirit and the ancestors. Trees are more than mere trees; the sky is more than what we see. There is more to plants and animals than we see with our eyes. Everything in the universe is a language of Life and an expression of Life. Therefore they are sacred and holy.

If you want to know how beautiful the mountains and the forests are, listen to their language. If you want to hear the language of Life, listen to the creatures. To be alive is to hear the echoes of life in forests, mountains, oceans, animals, the universe and in every human being.

For us Africans, everything and every person is a duality. Our world is not an either/or world. Our world is a both/and world. No good without bad, no life without death, no happiness without sorrow, no strength without weakness, no pride without shame and no pleasure without pain. Life is not opposed to death. Rather, life is life and death. The rain that waters our farms and wets the hot ground also brought the flood that drowned our goats and leaked through the roofs of our homes. The eyes with which we see and admire our loved ones also rain tears for them when they die. Today we wail, tomorrow we laugh. Today we fight, tomorrow we play together. Life is a rhythmic movement and an interaction between opposites. The rhythm of night and day, life and death, joy and sorrow, white and black, failure and success. It is by getting into this rhythm and fitting oneself into it, that one learns to live. He or she who would live a full, forceful life had better learn to fit him or herself into the rhythm of life. The riddles of life cannot be solved by dualism, by separating life from death, joy from sorrow and sickness from health. Rhythm is the means by which we understand and interpret life.

It often happens at the beginning of a new century that people suddenly discover that indeed, the long awaited new century has come, that the world has not ended as expected, that life continues (eternally) as usual and that no race has been wiped out. They then become discouraged and confused. Many stop going to church and may even doubt the existence of God. But what really is the meaning of the end of the world? Is God going to destroy the hills, the mountains, plants and animals? What sins have they committed? Is it not us human beings who have sinned? We really need to understand more deeply the meaning of the end of the world? Do not be surprised if in the first decade of the new century, that Churches are no longer filled with people; our seminaries and convents may no longer be filled with young men and women. Many so-called prophets may vanish. That would be the time to know who is a believer. When the son of man returns, will he find any faith on earth?

## The End is the Beginning

In the beginning, there was Life. Life has a beginning; therefore it must have an end. But the end is only a beginning. The beginning is the end. Therefore there is no end and no beginning, except in human thinking. For the end and the beginning are one. How can you prepare to meet God tomorrow when you have not learnt to meet God today? If God is not in your present moment, how can God be in your future moments?

It is amazing how the people of today crave for material power, forgetting that power in the real sense, is spiritual. We hear about ballistic missiles, atomic bombs, automatic rifles, and chemical weapons, which can wipe out the human race. It must be made known to the world that love is the greatest force in the world. What is the atomic bomb? A mere physical instrument, not to be compared with the spiritual energy that holds the world in existence.

In the beginning, God created heaven and earth. God created man and woman and put them in the garden, filled with beautiful plants and animals. In the beginning man and woman lived in harmony with the universe. They lived in perfect health of mind and body. They lived on the most natural and perfect food on earth, fruits and vegetables.

In the beginning our ancestors lived with only one consciousness. That is, the consciousness of God. They did not make a sharp division between the mind and body, spirit and soul, this world and beyond. They were aware only of the one reality-God, Life and Love. Adam and Eve allowed themselves to be deceived by the serpent. They ate the forbidden fruit and their eyes were opened. They were no longer at ease and they became diseased. They became alienated from themselves, from nature and from God. This alienation is what we call sin. They no longer saw themselves as part of the universe.

They began to relate to nature as something to exploit and use. Today, we are called upon to go back to nature. "Israel, come back to your God," says the prophet Isaiah. This same call is directed to the people of today. Come back to nature, for nature is spiritual. Come back to your God. Remember who you are. You are dust and unto dust you shall return. Air pollution, atomic energy, test tube babies, ballistic missiles, motor cars, and computers; is that what you call progress?

We need a new beginning. A new way of relating to one another and to the universe. This new relationship requires a new way of thinking, a new way of looking at the world, and a new understanding of the human person. Cultivate an attitude of respect and reverence for things and people. Let your mind be open to the voice of the Spirit. Often, you are full of yourself, your own ideas, your plans, and your beliefs. You strive to possess, to acquire, to control, to dominate and to exploit. Such attitudes lead to ignorance, not knowledge. Learn to be still, observe and admire the beauty of nature. If you look deeply enough, she will speak to you, for nature is alive. You are part of nature and to know nature is to know yourself.

## *The Road to Wholeness*

In 1999, I participated in a workshop on natural medicine. The workshop took place in the remote village of Ikposogye in the Obi Local Government Area of Nassarawa State, Nigeria. In attendance were nurses, midwives, farmers and housewives attending from different parts of the world like Germany, France, Switzerland and Nigeria. For one full week, this group of about forty men and women lived together, ate together, danced together, had discussions together, tilled the soil together and cleared bushes together. We emphasized on the spread of diseases all over Africa and diseases that can be cured by plants growing around us. We concluded that the truth about natural medicine should not be allowed to die. We must tell our fellow brothers and sisters to wake up from their slumber and be liberated.

Natural medicine is not just about increasing the physical life force of an individual. It is a call to break loose the chains of ignorance and mental slavery and become what we are meant to be. We have been told that our modern society is a materialistic and irreligious society, and that we are living in a Godless and devilish age. But is that really so? Has human nature changed? Why is it that in our so-called Godless and atheistic age, books on spirituality and mysticism are bestsellers? Young people all over the world are flocking to the East to learn about mysticism and contemplation. It seems to me that behind the so-called materialism and individualism of modern men and women lays a deeper desire for transcendence and holiness for God. Today's men and women of good will are no longer content with obeying dogmas or memorizing catechism. They want a living and personal encounter with the vital God. This desire and longing is a grace. If Christianity does not respond adequately to this need of men and women, how can it be relevant? "Of what use is salt that has lost its taste?" Is this really a Godless age? I do not think so. God is very much alive in the world. God is in Rwanda, and in Burundi. God is very much with us. The world is thirsty for God. Humanity is hungry for God. But, alas, we seek God in the wrong way. We look for God in the wrong places. That is the heart of the problem.

### The Hunger of the World

We have only one problem . . . the lack of love. Our problem is not the lack of power, or the lack of leadership, nor the lack of money. Our problem is the lack of love. And the only solution to all our problems is love. The world is sick due to the lack of that love. The fruits of this lack of love are divisions, strife and violence. Look around you. What do you see? Angry faces, hungry stomachs, broken families, and warring nations. The image one gets is that of a people who are not at peace within themselves or with one another. And because we are not at peace within ourselves we continue to inflict more and more pain on one another. How can you give peace to someone else when you do not have peace within yourself? How can there be peace in the world when there is no peace in the human heart?

### Our Real Need

The world does not need any more computers, or more cars, or more machines, or new political and economic system. What the world really needs is love. There is a tendency in our time to draw a sharp line between the "developed" and "underdeveloped" people of the earth. The "developed" people are the people of Western Europe and Northern America. They are the world changers, with a high level of technological advancement and superior technical knowledge and skills. The "underdeveloped" people are the people of Africa, Asia and Latin America. These people are supposedly "backward and lack inventiveness." They are passive receivers of western technology and civilization; hence they are referred to as the third world. Behind this division lies a false concept of progress, and an arrogant concept of western civilization as the ideal model of civilization. Serious minded people all over the world are asking, why is it that despite the high growth in technology and scientific knowledge and industrialization, as well as improved standard of living in the so called developed or rich countries, that cases of suicide, violence, depression and meaninglessness still abound? The biblical saying: "What does it profit a man if he gains the whole world but losses his own soul?" has become a modern maxim.

The economy of the Third World countries is utterly at the mercy of the First World countries. In the health sector, the people of the Third world spend their life earnings on importing drugs made of chemicals from trees that are growing in their backyards. African doctors and nurses are trained in the western way of healing, while they detest their own traditional health system that sustained them in their childhood. The results are that the nation continues to grow poorer and dependent on imported goods. Herbal medicine is a call to fight against all forms of exploitation of the poor by the rich as Christ did, and against all forms of hypocrisy, deceit and dishonesty.

## *What is Holiness?*

Holiness is a state of union with God, oneself and with others. Others include your fellow human beings as well as plants, animals and indeed the whole of creation. When you discover that you are not just anybody or just a spirit, but a complete and whole person, then you will discover the meaning of holiness. Your body is you, yet you are not your body; yet you are more than your body. Your body makes you manifest. Your body says a lot about you, your reality, and your personality.

The holy person is the one who has discovered the balance between the physical, the psychological and the spiritual. Some people are spiritually well but psychologically sick. Some are psychologically all right but are sick in spirit. What we call sickness is the physical manifestation of the imbalance between the spiritual and the psychological.

## *The Root of Disease*

When I was a child my grandmother used to tell me that plants, palm trees, animals, mountains and forest could talk. I would begin to look around and stretch my ears, but I would hear nothing. So I asked my mother, "How can palm trees, the Iroko tree, and animals talk? Are they human beings?" She would reply, "There is more to seeing than what you see. There is more to hearing than what you hear." Yes, it is true that the palm trees can talk, the forest can dance, the animals can speak, but we do not hear and we do not see. In our pursuit of material comfort and material wealth, we have lost touch with ourselves. We have been carried away by the philosophy of the modern world, which tells us that the goal of life is to be rich, to be comfortable, to be famous, to search for wholeness, for personal development to seek after material things. And the more material things we possess, the unhappy we will become, because this material things cannot give us lasting security and peace. The society says; be rich, have pleasure, obtain power, be famous, for these are goals of life. The false conception of life, of all reality is the root of all diseases. Having imbibed the mechanistic world view, which sees natural things as mere objects to be exploited and the human body as a mere object of pleasure, we eat what we like, drink anything that comes our way and live as we want. The result of this is disease. We are no longer at ease. The illusion that science and technology can provide solutions to all our problems is gradually being shattered. Why is it that despite the technological advancement of America and Japan, the industrial revolution of Europe and the wonderful scientific breakthrough of our modern world, more and more people still die of "incurable" illness?

### The Road to Wholeness

To be holy is to be whole, and to be whole is to be a full and complete person, fully alive. The holy man or woman is never an individual. He or she is a person. An individual is opposed to a person. An individual does his or her own thing, goes his or her way and does not think of others. But a person is always thinking about others. He cannot define himself or herself except in relation to others. He or she is a person because of others. To be a person, is to be molded into the image of the blessed trinity. The Father is a Father because of the Son. Just as the Son is a Son because of the Father, and the Spirit is a Spirit because of the union of the Father with the Son. The road to wholeness is openness and trust. Openness is to listen and be ready to change. The trust is to take the risk of loving my neighbor as myself, to face the truth about myself and about others.

## Identity

*Go to the ancestral shrine*
*The Sacred groove in your chest*
*And here again the silent echoes*
*of the Ancestors' voices calling*
*Calling you to be awake, to arise*
*Shake off the shackles of inferiority*
*O sons and daughters of Africa*
*Face the void*
*Love the darkness*
*Go to the ancestral shrine*
*The Sacred groove in your chest*
*And hear again the silent echoes*
*of the Ancestors' voice*
*Calling you to be awake, to arise*

*For you can transform the earth*
*Only when you discover*
*Who you are.*

# CHAPTER TWO

# AFRICAN MEDICAL TRADITION

The origin and evolution of healing as a special skill long antedates other important human inventions such as agriculture and animal domestication and might as well deserve consideration as 'the oldest profession', says Charles Finch.

Hippocrates is customarily regarded as the "father of Medicine". When in 1930 J.H. Breasted translated the Edwin Smith papyrus, which antedates Hippocrates by over 2500 years, it became clear that Imhotep, an African, not Hippocrates, a Greek, is the real "father of medicine". The excavated Ebers papyri and the Edwin Smith papyrus are the most important medical textbooks of ancient Egypt, now known as the Ebers papyrus and the Edwin Smith papyrus. They date back to pre-pyramid times, over 4000 years ago.

Imhotep was adviser to the Pharaoh Djoser. A statesman, designer and builder of the world's first great edifice in stone, the step-pyramid of Saggara. Hippocrates was said to have descended from a long line of "Asclepiads", that is, devotees of the Greek healing god Asclepios, often identified with Imhotep.

Imhotep's father was Kanofer, a distinguished architect in the service of Pharaoh. His mother was Khreduankh, from Mende. Although he served and excelled as prime minister, Chief Scribe, ritualist and architect under the Pharaoh Djoser of the 3rd dynasty, Imhotep's gifts as a physician overshadowed all the others.

Hippocratic medicine had direct antecedents in Egyptian medicine. The Egyptians were writing medical textbooks as early as 5000 years ago. Out of the hundreds and thousands of papyri that may have been written, we are lucky to have at least 10, which give us a window into medical practice among those ancient Africans. The city-state of Athens used to import Egyptian physicians, as did most of the Kingdoms of the Near East. The "Magico-spiritual" and rational elements intermingle in Egyptian medicine. Healing has a psychic base. Today, modern medicine concedes that as much as 60% of illness has a psychic base and the 'placebo' effect of modern medicine arises from this.

The dissemination of medical knowledge was often limited to a few families, though others who show enough talent can be allowed to practice. The physician was highly respected, and is referred to as Hakim, [wise man or philosopher]. Doctors had their own boats and traveled the Nile to treat patients.

Rulers surrounded themselves with physicians to ensure they are well taken care of in case of illness. Medical cures ranged from the use of potent speech [incantation or magico-spiritual element] to the more preventive and rational diagnosis based on ancient Egyptian medical practices. Egyptian medical enterprise flowed across Rome and the rest of Europe, where it was modified over many centuries.

There were three routes to becoming a skilled physician in the medieval period. The first is through tutorship by ones parents. Sons and daughters of learned physicians often learned the profession from their father, and medicine might become a family's major professions for generations.

The second method is through self-teaching. There is evidence that students taught themselves by compiling a list of medical texts, which were then read until they were satisfied that their contents had been learned. The major pitfall of this method is that the student may misinterpret certain scientific terms in a way different from the intended meaning. That notwithstanding, successful doctors did come from this tradition.

The third method is that a student entered the medical profession through classes in hospitals or medical schools. Long before hospitals emerged in the Christian world, it already was highly regarded in the Islamic world where it reached a high degree of sophistication and was opened to practitioners of all faith. The earliest documented hospital was built at Baghdad, Iraq, by Harun al-Rashid [786-809].

The tradition of medical specialization is said to originate with the Egyptian ancient medical system. There were specialists who treated the different parts of the body: eyes, head, teeth, intestines etc. This tradition of specialization seemed to have disappeared for some centuries until it came back again in the 4th century BC. Once again this tradition disappeared around 30 BC and did not resurface until the 20th century.

Skulls found from ancient Egyptian graves indicated that they practiced trephination. This operation is forerunner of neurosurgery, and involves boring a hole through the skull to the outer covering of the brain to remove fragments from a skull fracture compressing the brain, to treat epilepsy and also headache.

### Medicine in sub-Saharan Africa

Why, one would ask, did the Egyptian medical expertise and sophistication, not spread to sub-Saharan Africa? The reason is that external invasions after 661BC caused the Egyptian officials to look northward towards Europe rather than the south. Thus trade in material goods and culture and medical knowledge was only trans-Mediterranean. Added to this is the factor of the famine and dry phase of c. 2500BC that created the Sahara desert and cause the Negroid cultures of middle Africa to move southwards. This effectively isolated sub-Saharan Africa from the scientific changes occurring in the Mediterranean basin.

Sub-Saharan African, with the exemption of Ethiopia, was predominantly non-literate until the 11th century AD when Islam introduced Arabic literacy into the western Sudan.

That literacy came late into sub-Saharan Africa does not mean that it has no history. In fact, some of the best ideas in the history of human thought were the earliest, yet most histories of ideas ignore them. This is due to the wrong assumption that history started with the invention of writing, thereby leaving out the ideas of our earliest ancestors. But most societies, for most of history, have esteemed oral tradition more highly than writing. Their ideas are inscribed in other ways—left in the fragments of material culture for archaeologists to unearth, or buried deep in modern minds for psychologists to excavate, or preserved in later ages by traditional societies, where anthropologists are sometimes able to elicit them.

Secondly, some people's prejudice make them suppose that there are no ideas worth the name in the minds of the ancients, whom they called 'primitive' or 'salvage', mired in "pre-logical" thought, or retarded by magic or myth. However, there has not been any evidence of any change in human brain capacity or in human intelligence since over 30,000 years ago.

Medical practice in sub-Saharan Africa is a combination of the magical, the mythical, the spiritual and the scientific. In Africa, a human being is a person, not just an individual. An individual is one who is on his own, who does his own thing, goes his own way and separates himself from others. He has a 'soul', a 'mind' and a 'body', all of which are distinct and at times opposed. A person, on the other hand, is a being who exists with and for others. A person is a person with and because of others. A person cannot define himself except in relation to others.

African medicine does not just involve herbs. In African medicine, the use of animal parts, music, sacred chants, potent speech, dance and touch are prominent. In many parts of Africa, animal parts such as liver, kidney, gall bladder, and gizzard are burnt to ashes and used as part of herbal ingredients for various illnesses. For example, cow tail and liver burnt to ashes is said to be good remedy for diabetes. An energetic analysis of these animal parts show that these organs are high vibratory organs with high electromagnetic fields, and taking them as medicine is a good way of transmitting these energy waves to the diseased organs.

Legend has it that the earliest form of healing in Africa is vibrational healing. As an example among many others, the Yoruba of western Nigeria have a highly developed system of vibratory healing. The founding father of African-Yoruba medical practice is a man called Orunmila, who, like many other African heroes, was deified, or, to use a more technical term, immortalized. Just as European scientists such as Galileo, Faraday, Newton, Descartes and Einstein, have been immortalized in our memories, so also do Africa heroes deserve to be remembered and appreciated not just by Africans but by the world.

Even though Orunmila is regarded as the founding father of African-Yoruba medicine, the title of 'father of Yoruba medicine' is accorded a man called Osanyin. Osanyin had the gift of communicating with plants. He could so attuned himself to the energy field of plants that through his perception of the vibration of these plants, gain knowledge of their uses. As a young man, whenever he was sent to the farm, he would refuse to cut any grass because he was psychically sensitive to nature, and was aware of the usefulness of each plant.

Osanyin did not just have knowledge of herbs. He also knew how to use the energy of plants to effect changes in human bodily conditions. This he did through the chanting of sacred chants or potent speech. Osanyin taught that one way to attune oneself to the energy waves of plants is to learn their names and pronounce them audibly. African tradition is an oral tradition, and so pride of place is given to memory work and careful use of words. As a child grows up, they are taught how to use words and to avoid saying certain words that may attract a negative spirit. Rhythm governs words, discussions and daily life as a whole. By rhythmic combination of words, Africans get themselves attuned to universal cosmic vibrations and so are able to maintain balance in their lives. This explains why music permeates and defines every aspect of the daily lives of Africans. When going to the stream to fetch water, children chant. When working in the farm, farmers sing. When eating, the eaters follow a rhythmic pattern of washing hands, putting the food in their mouths, chewing and drinking. When nursing, mothers never cease to sing lullabies. In times of danger, Africans sing or recite sacred mantras to ward off danger.

Sickness is believed to be as a result of disharmony between the physical and the spiritual. The aim of the priest-physician is to restore this harmony. To do this, he had to find out what causes the disharmony. He uses different diagnostic tools to find this out: the oracle, like the Ifa Oracle of the Yoruba, or counselling with the sick. Having diagnosed what the problem is, the next thing is the treatment. Treatment could involve rituals, prayers, confession of one's guilt if one has offended the 'gods'. It could also involve the preparation of herbs, animal parts as medicine.

Various methods are used to detect the medicinal values of herbs. In traditional African societies, and indeed in other parts of the world, people look at the colour and shape as well as the location of a plant to get an insight into its use and importance. This is called the theory of signatures. They believe that plants grow in any specific area because there is a need for them. Herbs that grow on mountains are believed to be good for the respiratory system-lungs, bronchi, nostrils and the nervous system. They cure high blood pressure as well as pneumonia. Herbs that grow in water are regarded as very medicinal. In the first place, they are almost always edible, since poisonous herbs very rarely grow in water. They are good for the circulatory system and help in repairing the liver and the kidney, two vital organs in the body. Herbs that grow in water are believed to be good for treating all forms of infertility in both men and women. For the treatment of impotence, water herbs are very effective.

Herbs that grow close to the soil are believed to be good for digestive and circulatory problems. Since they are close to the ground, the mineral content is high, and so is good for the bones and blood. Those who suffer from anaemia would find these herbs useful. Granted that the theory of signatures is not always true, it is amazing to see how much of the insights of the ancients have been confirmed by modern science as true.

From time to time, traditional healers prescribe that certain herbs be harvested only at a certain time of the day. Sometimes they insist that certain plants should be harvested before sunrise, some after sunset. At times they go out themselves in the middle of the night to collect some herbs. This practice in itself is scientifically correct. In the night, when the sun has already transverse the earth and has set for the day, the chemical compounds in many plants, especially trees, settle down to the roots of the trees. In order to get the best out of these roots then, it is advisable to harvest them at sunset, which in tropical countries begins from 5 in the evening. Now, somebody may come and tell you to do your harvesting at 10 pm rather than 5pm. They may tell you that the roots will not work for you unless you harvest them at 10 or 11pm or midnight. That extra detail or explanation is wrong against the background of our scientific knowledge. But the basic idea of harvesting the root at sunset is true.

When the sun begins to rise, plants, especially trees, draw up their chemical compounds and distribute them to the leaves and barks. By the middle of the day, these compounds are fully concentrated in the leaves of the plants. For this reason, the best time to harvest the leaves of medicinal plants is at midday, when the sun is about to reach its peak. By late afternoon, the chemical compounds in trees begin their downward journey back to the roots through the stems and barks. For this reason, the best time to collect the bark of a tree is late in the afternoon or in the evening, before sunset. Science has validated this practice of the ancients, which may at first appear to us as superstitious and mythical.

It is one of the sad aspects of the history of sub-Saharan Africa that we have no written records of the medical system of our ancestors. However, from the excavated surgical knives, the concoction jars, the carved statues of the various deities, we have a good idea of African medical practice in the ancient world, and we can now rewrite our history.

## Medicine in colonial Africa

When British, French and Portuguese explorers came to Sub-Saharan Africa, they found already established empires such as the Songhai, Mali, Hausa and Oyo empires with well-organised political and social systems, art works, sculptors [which now adorn the British museum]. Count Volney, friend of Benjamin Franklin, visited Egypt in 1783-1785. During the course if this travels he saw age-old monuments and temples half buried in the sand, which gave evidence of an advanced civilization, arts and the sciences. The gradual transition of Africa into a more scientific community and its emergence as a unique, independent cultural identity was abruptly interrupted by colonialism.

As the British conquered land after land, it also brought its physicians along to treat its administrators and troops. British administrators and troops die in their thousands due to diseases common in the tropics. Since Africans had immunities to some of the tropical diseases, it was decided to train Africans as doctors to assist British doctors in the imperial system. They adopted this system because there was no other arrangement that was preferable.

Imperial needs, then, led to the training of African physicians in the 18th and 19th centuries under incipient colonialism, under the auspices of the 'colonial medical service'.

The route to medical professionalism for those early Africans started at Edinburgh or Dublin. The Anglican Christian Missionary society selected 3 young adult Africans for training in Scottish Universities in 1854. In 1855, these 3 students were summoned to King's College, University of London. The Oldest, Samuel Campbell, was a Wolof. The Second, William Broughton Davies, was a Yoruba. The third, James Beale Horton, was an Igbo. These students were not sons of the elite but of manual labourers. They had grown up in Freetown, Sierra Leone, which had a population of one hundred and fifty thousand and European population of 150.

They were well educated in music, mathematics, the Greek and Roman classics, and in geography. Their manners and intellectual habits were moulded in accordance with those of the English middle class. However, Samuel Campbell could not cope with the sudden change in weather, and suffered severe cold and pneumonia, and had to return home. Within a short time of his arrival back in Freetown, he died of bronchitis in 1855. Davies fell ill but survived and completed his course. Horton coped very well with the weather and won top honours in his class and was soon made a member of King's college medical society. Both Horton and Davies passed the qualifying exams earning membership in the Royal College of Surgeons [MRCS] in 1858 and were given the licentiate in medicine. Horton and David proceeded to Scotland for their MD in medicine [equivalent to a PhD]. While a student Horton took the name Africanus as a sign of pride in his African ancestry. They both returned to Sierra Leone in 1859, the same year that epidemics of yellow fever, measles and smallpox had killed half the European population in West Africa.

Horton became a very active and successful surgeon, scientist, soldier, banker, businessman and a political thinker. Infact, Horton is seen as one of the founders of African nationalism. He is the author of numerous books which include *West African Countries and Peoples* [1868] and *The Diseases of Tropical Climates and Their Treatment* [1874].

Unlike most western-trained African doctors who deprecated indigenous medical practice, leading to a decline in herbal medicine and spiritual healing, Horton advocated the integration of traditional and western medicine in the treatment of disease and probably he was among the earliest to do so. Horton's MD thesis of 1859 at Edinburgh discusses how bark from the mangrove tree was used in the treatment of fevers in Gambia and how the leaves of the castor oil plant helped to boost the secretion of breast milk among women of the Cape Verde Islands. In Sierra Leone, Horton described how the citrus medicine was used to treat seasickness and that the unripe pawpaw (Carica papaya) was useful in expelling worms. During his tenure as an army doctor in the Gold Coast, Horton reported how the use of tinctures from the herbal 'assafetida was useful in curing guinea worm infections.

Over the past ten years, I have worked with a number of western-trained medical practitioners who are passionate about Traditional Medicine and are researching into herbal remedies with the intention of incorporating them into their practice. I salute the courage and creativity of these doctors and ask others who are either too lazy to research or too proud to acknowledge the efficacy of herbal medicine to follow in the footsteps of Dr. Horton and dare to be different! If it works, prove it. And if it is proven, why not accept it and incorporate it into your practice. If that is not science, then I wonder what science is.

Despite the fact that they attended the same medical school and passed through the same training, the medical officers of the British middle class generally refused to regard the Africans as their peers and resented their presence. White racial prejudices were reinforced by theories like polygenesis, which held that whites and blacks were not really of the same human species, having evolved from different ancestors. These attitudes were a big barrier to progress for the African doctors. African doctors were not allowed to treat White patients, especially white women.

To the medical elite, university training provided for a more powerful lobbying position toward influencing the state. Medical training provided a way for the medical elites to distinguish themselves from, and seek preferential treatment over their traditional competitors-apothecaries, grocers, barbers and the lay African practitioners. As matters turned out, the colonial administrators did nothing to alter this situation, a legacy which still hampers health care delivery in independent Africa.

Two health systems prevailed: the emerging African elite patronized medical doctors in the cities, but in the urban, slums and rural peripheries. Traditional medicine remained dominant. The medical elite operated as if oblivious of the fact that a health system had been in place centuries earlier and made very little effort in applying their western analytical methods to study the existing traditional health systems in order to see if there are points of convergence. This led to an inter-professional conflict which persists till the present time.

British physicians refer to their African colleagues as "Native doctors" as distinct from "European doctors". Infact, the term "Native doctor" was the official colonial term for African doctors from the 1800s till independence. This term was greatly resented by the African doctors who went to the same school as the

Europeans and often scored distinctions, but were not allowed the same prestige as European doctors. The 'Native doctors' treated only blacks while Europeans doctors treated both whites and blacks. On no account was an African doctor allowed to examine or treat a white woman. It was presumed that African doctors were inherently inferior to European doctors, an idea which lingers till today even among Africans.

Because of their specialized educational training, doctors and lawyers were accepted in the elite circles and were taken seriously as political candidates. Their professional credentials lent them prestige and freed them from suspicions of corruption and nepotism that conventional politicians have always been subjected to. In response to the social needs of their time, 19th and 20th century doctors often left their medical practise, sometimes permanently, in order to be involved in the new dynamism of politics, nationalism and liberation struggle. In fact, the first political organization in Nigeria, the People's Union, was founded by medical doctors: John Randall [1855-1928] and Orisadipe Obasa [1863-1940] in Lagos. In Cote d'Ivoire, Dr. Felix Houphouet-Boigny was life president. Dr. Milton Morgai became first prime minister of Sierra Leone republic in 1961. Dr. Hastings Kamuzu led Malawi to independence in the early 1960s and became the life president. In the 1970s the late president Samora Moises Machel, a nurse, won independence for Mozambique from the Portuguese while Dr. Ayostinho Neto led Angola to independence in the same era. In Nigeria, Dr. Ishaya Audu, a paediatrician, served as foreign secretary in the new republic of Nigeria.

The Yaba Medical Training College is the first medical school in Nigeria. It started in October 1930 as a school for training medical assistants, not physicians, and awarded diplomas which were given recognition by the Royal College of Surgeons, England. In 1948 the Yaba School began a transfer and merger with the new University College of Ibadan. The Ibadan University College graduated its first medical class in November 1960. With special permission from London, 13 students received the MB and Bsc degrees in medicine. Among them was Dr. Adelola Adeloye, the well-known medical historian, author of *"African Pioneers of Modern Medicine. Nigerian Doctors of the Nineteenth Century.*

### Medicine in post-colonial Africa

Since the Christian missionaries operated under the auspices of Colonial masters, Africans came to identify colonialism with Christianity. Western medicine was called 'Christian medicine', while African traditional Medicine was called 'Pagan medicine'. What this means is that to be a convert, one must 'renounce the devil and all its establishments', which includes traditional or pagan medicine. Medical doctors were called 'Christian doctors' or 'white doctors' [the doctor's white garment symbolises purity and cleanliness], while traditional healers were called 'pagan doctors'. The term 'native doctor', which was originally used by western physicians to describe their African colleagues until independence, was used to describe traditional healers as from the mid-1960s till date. It is ironical that African medical doctors who complained bitterly about the arrogant attitudes of their white colleagues exhibited the same arrogant and superior attitudes to traditional healers and saw them as competitors rather than as collaborators.

After independence, government policies maintained the inherited colonial structure and made very little effort to develop African traditional medicine. Because of their training, African doctors could not relate in any way to traditional healers who were regarded as unlettered, pagan and often crude and unhygienic in their way of treating people. Because of their specialised training, African doctors saw themselves as an enlightened, educated, civilised and an elite species of health care providers.

It is important to note that Western medicine in the 19th century is closer to Traditional Medicine than it is today. Western medicine laid emphasis on mixtures mainly from herbal extracts. The Europeans mixed their own drugs and measured them into brown bottles to preserve their potency. Huge extracts from the root of the Brazilian plant *ipecacuanha* were ordered to cure cough, a drug that remains one of the strongest cough ingredients till today. Opium was also used to treat sick people. Yet, the European pharmacists and physicians had no intention of working with traditional healers.

Following this tradition, African doctors sought to superimpose medical practices and experiences learned outside of Africa on communities that had little or no respect for western values. In order to survive, they had to 'fight' the traditional healers and win over their patients by exposing their ignorance of physiology and anatomy. It was clear that unless the status of the traditional healers was diminished, the people will continue to patronize them, thereby making the financial survival of doctors in private practice difficult.

On the other hand, African healers would direct their patients to the hospitals when their treatment failed, and it did not take long before the effectiveness of western medicine became recognized among the communities. The people's confidence in western medicine grew following the development of sulfa drugs in the mid-1930s, and antibiotics in World War II, when physicians were able to attack most pathogenic bacteria effectively. One example is river blindness which decimated many populations in West Africa. By the 1950s drugs for this sickness had been found. This and other inventions humiliated traditional healers who suffered diminished status in the eyes of African patients, while African Medical doctors enjoyed increased status.

Today, Africa is faced with the challenge of re-understanding, re-inventing, re-expressing ancient knowledge [indigenous knowledge] in the light of modern scientific knowledge [exogenous]. This requires a synergy of both systems. In order to become global, one must first of all *be local*. While the indigenous needs the exogenous to rise to global integrity, the fact remains that the exogenous loses its substance and transformative power without the indigenous. For example, while there has been a rapid, breathtaking technological innovation in medicine, there has not been a corresponding change in medical curriculum in Nigerian universities. That means that medical curriculum in Nigerian universities has undergone very minimal change in the past 30 years. A course in business administration, for example, is done the same way as it is done in, say, an American university, as if the student is an American. A law curriculum is arranged in such a way that pre-eminence is given to the study of laws that originated in Europe. The point is that when there is no proper synergy between the indigenous and exogenous, education becomes artificial and insubstantial. This is why we fail to see how absurd it is that a Nigerian lawyer, or a laboratory scientist, or a bank manager or medical practitioner is expected to observe a certain dress code [suited to European climate] without reference to the weather condition of the place where they live.

For African medicine, the future lies in the ability to be opened to the challenges of globalization through proper documentation, analysis and research. While countries like China and India have already invaded the global herbal market like a colossus, Nigeria is still busy discussing whether herbal medicine is a good source of health care or not. While the global market for Herbal medicine is estimated to be 60 billion dollars, African professionals are busy attending seminars to convince them of the efficacy of herbal medicine. And while Chinese medical doctors, botanists, pharmacists and other scientists are all united in the development of their traditional medicine into a global transformative venture, Nigerian scientists are standing by the ring-side complaining about the attitude of charlatans and quacks. A better approach is to join hands in correcting the perceived weaknesses and mistakes of our traditional medicine, and help transform it into a globally acceptable enterprise.

# CHAPTER THREE

# HERBAL MEDICINE AND THE REVIVAL OF AFRICAN CIVILIZATION

It is said that humanity is going through the most fertile, creative, productive and fruitful period of history. Contemporary civilization is the greatest producer of wealth, affluence, prosperity and 'development'. Ironically, it is also the producer of the greatest pollution, destruction, poverty, hunger, violence, hatred and inequality between humans. Many 'developed' countries are underdeveloped in many ways, while many developing countries are really not developing.

While the north is struggling with negative effects of overdevelopment, mis-development or mal-development, Africa is struggling with the negative effects of slow or no development. The north is excessively rich, Africa is excessively poor.

Both poverty and wealth put pressure on the resource bases of the world. The rich contribute to damaging the earth through excessive greed, consumerism and unsustainable lifestyle. The poor also damage the earth through bush burning, cutting down valuable trees without any plan to replace them by cultivation, selling rare animal parts all in a bid to raise some money to feed. Poverty is as bad as excessive wealth. Both over-development and under-development are incompatible with sustainable development. Europe and America are well-developed but at a costly price. Biodiversity loss and climate change have resulted in agricultural intensification and greenhouse emissions.

### A look at Asia

China's Gross Domestic Product [GDP] has grown by over 10% in the past 5 years, while India's has grown by 8-9%. More than 500 million people in China have been lifted out of poverty in the past 25 years. Vietnam's GDP has grown more than 8% per year for the past 3 years. In 1976, Malaysia's poverty rate was 50% (same as Nigeria]. Today, it is said to be less than 5%. In 1993, Vietnam's poverty level was nearly 60%, now it is under 20%. Economics project that if current trends continue, Asian's portion of global GDP will rise from 30% today to 50% by 2040.

However, Asia's growth has come with a price. Asia is in danger of losing up to 75% of its forests and 40% of its biodiversity this century. Already, in the past 25years, Asia lost one-half of its forests, degraded one-third of its agricultural land and became home to 13 of the world's 15 most polluted cities, according to the institute of Global Environmental strategies in Japan. As India's growing number of middle class family increased in numbers and wealth, it has caused an increase in demand for foodstuffs, and its production capacity of agriculture can't meet the demand. Similar trends are taking place in Indonesia, Philippines, Vietnam and Brazil.

## *A look at Africa*

Looking at Africa, what is obvious is not the growth of basic and mature engineering, automation, post-harvest preservation, food processing and packaging technologies, infrastructural developments, social amenities, oil management technology and water technology, all of which are vital for poverty eradication. Rather, what is more evident is the spread of Dogmatic/religious knowledge, extraordinary sprouting of churches, Pentecostalism and piety, which demands dogmatic and unquestioning submission to revealed 'truths', and discouragement of reason, dissidence and logic. What is outwardly evident to a traveler in Nigeria, for example, are not sites of new manufacturing factories, sprouting of small scale industries or centers of excellence for research and information technology. The only visible activities seem to be in the religious sphere, where new, gigantic churches are being constructed, millions of new small churches mushrooming, huge bill-boards and media advertisements of miracle crusades, prosperity vigils and 'spiritual war'.

Excessive religionism and spiritualism may be one of the greatest obstacles to progress of African nations. And the greatest challenge facing Africa today may well be her ability to cultivate a mindset steeped in chemistry, mathematics and physics and still maintain a reasonable and balanced approach to religion.

The term development, as used in this work, refers to the ability of nations to order the society in such a way that there is order, basic amenities such as water, housing, security, road and energy.

Viewed in this sense, it is true that many African countries have never experienced 'development' or modernity.

Many African nations are yet to upgrade, renew and evolve their knowledge bases. They find a lazy and easy excuse in referring to times past, the 'good old days', to ancient ways of life that are not compatible with modern realities. Others blame colonialism, Capitalism, Civilisation or modernity. It is true that we were once enslaved; it is true that some capitalist foreigners invaded our land and ruled over us, and exploited our natural resources for selfish gains. But were we the only race that was so colonised? And how long shall we continue to blame other people for our woes? Is it not time we courageously face our problems and see them as challenges for growth? When a man in faraway Spain says something derogatory about a black man, we all rightly stand up in protest against his racist tendencies. But why wouldn't we also wage war against the tribalist in each of us, among our own kith and kin?

### Science without substance

European colonizers did not introduce science into their overseas territories because they wanted their subjects to become scientists. Their aim was rather to teach *peripheral science*, an impoverished science deprived of an inner qualitative element that could give rise to integral research. Thus science in the colonies was marked by theoretical emptiness. First there is the frantic accumulation of facts and data, which begins the scientific enquiry. And then followed the last stage, which is the application of theoretical findings to practical issues. But the most important stage, the stage that comes between them, was lacking. This middle stage, the interpretation of raw information, the theoretical processing of the data collected, and the production of those particular utterances which we call scientific statements, took place in the colonizers' home countries. Deprived of the will to transform, peripheral science lacked the very context, character and powers of co-creation that made capitalist and scientific endeavours productive in the colonizers' own country.

European research in Africa was performed to benefit the colonialists or the mother country. Africans rarely advanced beyond assistants. Moreover, education for Africans imbued them with contempt of manual labor. Consequently they eschewed farming and generally did not apply their knowledge to make greatly needed improvements in the areas of agriculture, medicine, engineering, architecture etc. The African landscape is today filled with young university graduates who are desperately looking for white-collar jobs. Employment in the banking industry or legal profession is the dream of most African graduates. Farming, mechanics, construction are regarded as dirty jobs and have no prestige in the society. University education, as it is constituted in Africa today, is geared towards producing graduates who are *job seekers* rather than *job creators* or entrepreneurs.

What is needed in the developing world today, especially in Africa, is not just to apply traditional knowledge in agriculture or medicine or architecture while continuing to import from the west scientific and managerial methods that are poorly understood and mastered by the local users. African governments are often tempted to prolong the length of time students spend in school because they believe that the longer time they spend in school the more educated they become. Similarly, African governments mistakenly think that the way forward is to import more knowledge into their countries. However, what is really needed is to help the people and their elite to capitalize and master the existing knowledge, whether indigenous or not, and develop new knowledge in a continual process of *uninterrupted creativity*, while applying the findings in a systematic and responsible way to improve their own quality of life. This is our road to greatness. We must create our own systems or be forever enslaved in other people's. The ball is in our court.

## Killing the earth

Recently, I got an invitation to deliver a lecture at a proposed workshop on preserving our earth. The idea of the workshop came from the fact that human beings have selfishly and greedily exploited the earth's resources in such a way that human existence is in jeopardy. Already, hundreds of thousands of plants and animals are said to be extinct, while the ozone layer has been severely affected, and the earth has become warmer than is normal. The Industrial Revolution that began in the middle of the 1700s brought a sharp increase in burning coal, which produces carbon dioxide, called a greenhouse gas. As a greenhouse gas it helps to heat up the air and therefore increases global climate temperatures. This is called the greenhouse effect. Humans have already increased the levels of carbon dioxide in the atmosphere by more than 30% since the beginning of the industrial revolution and the large-scale use of fossil fuels.

The issue of global warming or climate change and how to prevent and reduce it now tops the agenda of most international agencies, including the United Nations. These agencies are spending billions of dollars in sponsoring awareness programmes on global warming, and what we can do to reduce it. Not long ago I had written to an international development agency applying for sponsorship for a skill acquisition programme for the poor men and women of Ewu village where I reside. The response was clear and simple: we are not interested in such a programme. However, I was advised that if I change the theme of the programme to "Going Green', or "How to Reduce Global Warming', my application may be accepted. Point well understood: "He who pays the piper dictates the tune. If you want our money, say what we want you to say, think as we want you to think, act as we want you to act".

This manipulation is even more intense on the intercontinental level. The United nations have mandated the African Union [AU] to have as top on their agenda issues of global warming or climate change, or lose sponsorship for many of their programmes. In December 2008 at the UN sponsored African Union summit on climate change, African leaders were bluntly told that if they want continuous foreign aid, they must be actively involved in promoting among Africans an awareness of the dangers of global warming. In order words, African leaders should discourage mechanized mass agriculture, stop African hunters from killing animals, reduce their use of electricity [in Nigeria this is hardly available], and 'go green' [plant more trees, flowers]. Some African leaders are now asking why they should be compelled to sacrifice rapid economic growth for 'going green'. James Lovelock, a British scientist, stated categorically that the earth cannot sustain an industrialised Africa. Message: Africa should remain underdeveloped and technologically weak so that the rich north can continue to enjoy their opulence.

Meanwhile, in the United States and Canada, individuals release over 10,000 pounds of carbon dioxide [$CO_2$] per person per year. Heating and cooling systems in the US emit over 500 million tons of $CO_2$ into the atmosphere each year. While people in the rich countries decide which gas-consuming cars to buy, Africans are seeking firewood and charcoal to cook their meals [which the UN now discourages]. New York alone uses more gasoline in a week than the whole of Africa does in a year. There are more cars in Germany than in the whole of Africa. The US State of Texas alone, with a population of 30 million, emits more $CO_2$ than 93 developing countries added together, with a combined population of nearly one billion people.

## Can we heal the earth?

Now back to the proposed workshop earlier mentioned. The topic I am asked to speak on is: *Healing the earth*. I am asked to emphasis the fact that human beings have damaged the earth almost irredeemably, and we should do what we can to 'safe' mother earth, to heal and make her whole again. As I reflected on my topic, it dawned on me that human beings have yet to learn the lessons of history due to our sheer arrogance.

In the first place, what gave us the audacity to think that we can heal the earth? If the earth needs healing, who is the doctor? Looking at the natural order of things, who is really in need of healing, the earth or humanity? The earth is not in need of healing. It is humanity who is sick and needs healing. And we have no other healer than mother earth. Was our estrangement from the earth not the cause of our sickness? Rather than seeking to 'heal the earth', we should learn to live in harmony with the healing earth.

The mess in which inhumanity finds itself today was caused by a wrong understanding of knowledge and its role in human development. Firstly, we were led astray by the myth that with enough knowledge and technology [computers, digital machines, satellites, buttons, etc], we can rule the earth and control it. But the complexity of the earth and its life systems can never be safely managed. We can never master the complex functioning of atoms, protons, ions and electricity. With the help of technology, we have abused the earth and populated it with over six billion greedy individuals. What needs to be managed is not the earth, but human desires, economics, politics and communities.

### Between sanity and madness

There was an eighteenth century psychiatrist who developed an ingenious method of distinguishing the sane from the insane. He locked those to be diagnosed in a room with water taps on one side and a supply of mops and buckets on the other. He then turned on the taps: the mad ones ran for the mops and buckets while those he considered sane simply walked up to the tap and turned it off. The 'mop and bucket' mentality is so prevalent in our world today that it is taken to be the norm. Heavily dressed professionals and so called experts receive fat salaries for providing 'mop and bucket' solutions to problems of education, economics, governance, health and environment. Our society has failed to distinguish between cleverness and intelligence, between 'know-how' and 'know why'.

Recently, a governor of one of the Niger Delta states of Nigeria closed down the state school of Arts and Culture and converted it to a science school because, according to him, the state needs more of scientists than poets and artists. Could it be that our so-called modern society score high in cleverness but low in intelligence? Could it be that while human beings have been able to perform amazing technological feats, they are unable to solve their most basic human problems? Our over-emphasis on specialization has led to proliferation of 'experts' who can only think in one direction and lack a holistic view of life. They cannot see the link between finance and ecology, between mathematics and spirituality, between engineering and the sound of the ocean, between oil exploration and a healthy eco-system.

### The grand illusion

Our students passed out of universities with a distorted view of reality, of nature and of the cosmos. Some of these students score high in their examinations and are then regarded as 'experts'. They are seen as brilliant and clever. They have the technical knowhow but cannot ask the deeper questions of life. University education provides them with answers without knowing what the questions are.

One of the great illusions of our time is the myth that the purpose of education is to give students the means for upward mobility and success. Most students are brainwashed to think that the reason why they go to school is to get a career. And that the inevitable means is to acquire paper certificates. In Nigeria, students are ready to do anything from the bizarre to the weird and deadly in order to get certificates. Our society prides acquisition of degrees over holistic and integral development. The goal of education is not mastery of subject matter but mastery of one's person. The goal of education is not to stuff facts, techniques, methods and information into the students' mind but rather to teach them how to use ideas and knowledge to develop one's own personhood. Rather than see education as a means of personal development, most students see it as a step towards getting careers that will launch them into a so-called 'successful' life. Proper education should help students to find a decent calling or vocation, not just a career. A career is a job, a way to earn one's daily bread. It's a ticket to something else. A calling is about life, personhood, values and one's vocation and gift to the world. It comes out of one's inner convictions. A career can always be found in a calling, but hardly the other way round.

### Fragmented knowledge

Take the field of Medicine as an example. There are so many specializations: eye, nose, ear, bone, blood, teeth, brain, heart, skin, kidney, hair etc. For the purpose of teaching and analysis, it is alright to fragment an object into sections. But the problem is that we often forget to lead the students back to the fact that wholeness is the true nature of life. If a sick person has eye, nose, kidney and heart problems, they would have to visit five different 'specialists', as if they were some disjointed pieces of machine. Such sense of dichotomy does not promote healing but impacts negatively on the psychology of the sick. Knowledge based only on 'know-how' is knowing in fragments, knowing without discretion, without direction, without commitment.

Nature is characterized by integrity, beauty, stability and wholeness. Everything is connected with everything else. Nothing stands alone. The earth rotates round the sun in perfect equilibrium. If our earth had been a little bit closer to the sun, it would have been too hot for habitation. If on the other hand the earth had been a little bit further away from the sun, it would have been too cold for habitation. Human beings and plants exchange oxygen and carbon dioxide in such a balanced way that life can continue.

Today, the implication of human greed, pride and exploitation of the earth is manifesting in climate change, global warming, depletion of the ozone layers and extinction of thousands of species of plants and animals. Each day mother earth loses about 120 square miles of rain forest and at least 50 species of plants and animals. Not only that, at least 3000 tons of chlorofluoro-carbons and 20 million tons of carbon dioxide are added to the atmosphere, making it hotter, more fragile and less life-sustaining.

Humanity has attained technological height at the cost of the very things on which our future health and prosperity depend: climate stability, a balanced biocosm, a productive natural system, the beauty of nature and biological diversity.

For centuries, human beings lived under the illusion that with enough knowledge and technology, we can manage and control the earth. And for centuries, as new factories and industries produced more computers, electronics and machines, we thought we had succeeded in mastering the earth. We thought that a rapid increase in data, words, paper and technical details is equivalent to increase in knowledge and wisdom. The truth however, is that as we grew in technical knowledge, in 'know-how', we lost other kinds of knowledge: intelligence, which is characterized by ability to foresee the consequences of one's actions, wisdom and 'know-why'.

For humanity to survive, we must give up our arrogance and the misleading conception that western culture represents the pinnacle of human achievement. We need to learn how to be human. We need to learn to relate to the earth in a positive and productive way. The word humility is derived from the Latin *humus*, which means earth, ground, earthliness, humanness. To be human is to be humble, and see ourselves as part of, not the centre of, creation. To be human is to be healed by the healing earth. This is our challenge in the 21ˢᵗ century.

### *A new revolution*

There is a revolution taking place right now in the world. Call it a silent revolution if you like. It is a revolution that is redefining the world and our place in the planet earth. Men and women of goodwill in every corner of the earth are joining forces together to challenge and query the *status quo*, reclaiming our rights to a new, wholistic view of life.

Millions of groups, societies and organizations all over the world are working on the most salient issues of our day: climate change, poverty, deforestation, peace, water, hunger, conservation, human rights and Justice. This is the largest revolutionary movement the world has ever seen. Rather than control, it seeks connection. Rather than dominance, it strives to disperse concentration of power. It provides hope, support and meaning to billions of people in the world. Its power comes from ideas, not force.

When God made men and women, he gave them all they needed to be happy, to be whole, to be healthy: He gave us sunshine, water, air and the earth. But due to our greediness and selfishness, we began to exploit the earth, abuse it, destroy it, and treat it without respect. The result is crisis: economic crisis, mental crisis, social crisis, political crisis and climatic crisis.

We who are adults know that we have lost our childhood innocense, and we know that somehow, our happiness depends on regaining it. Somehow, we know that we have lost touch with nature, and somewhere deep in our hearts we know that we need to get in touch with nature. We human beings are the youngest occupants of this planet. Before we came, the plants were here. Before we came, the animals were here. Before we came, the oceans, the forests, the mountains were here. To survive, we must learn from them. And to learn from them, we must respect them.

### Together for better or for worse

The air we breathe is the same air inhaled by Jesus Christ, by the Blessed Virgin Mary, by Mohammed, and by the great scientists, philosophers and saints of the past. Their utterances, thoughts and breath are still present in the air molecules in which we are immersed. So long as we all breathe the same air, we will all remain bonded together, both the living and the dead. Viewed from this perspective, one can now see how scientific our Africans ancestors were when they asserted that only a thin line separates the spiritual from the physical, spirit from matter, life from death. The wisdom of the ancients is there in the molecules of the air around us, waiting to be tapped when we are open enough to perceive them. Our health, our life, our future, depends on the quality of the air around us. The rich, the poor, the sick, the healthy, black people, white people, we all breathe the same air. There is no separate air for different categories of people. At the end of the day, what we put into the air will come back to us, either as puritans or as poison.

The idea of the stranger, the unknown is an illusion. We are all linked together in a symbiotic cosmos. What affects one affects all. The internet has been a unifying force for different groups all over the world, both for good and for evil. On the positive side, it has given rise to the most powerful movement in the world: a coming together of men and women of goodwill fighting for their rights, fighting for the right to be human, to be free. On the negative side, it has provided a breeding ground for the Al Qaeda and many terrorists groups to unite, source for funds and maintain global linkage.

Nobody is destined to be poor, or to be sick. We have the right to challenge the *status quo*. Many people all over the world are challenging capitalism itself, a system that is based on intense greed, selfishness and deceit. A few privileged elite numbering a few thousands possess and acquired over 80% of world wealth and leave the remaining 5.5 billion people to scramble for the remaining 20%.

Millions of men and women from all parts of the world are coming together to remind us that it is our human greed and selfishness, rather than nuclear bombs, that constitute the greatest threat to human survival, human health and human peace. Humanity is sick and needs to be administered the medicine of justice, fairness, concern for others and respect for our symbiotic cosmos.

## Knowledge without local substance

Have you heard our young men discussing about football recently? They know the latest news on soccer in the English premier league. They can tell you when Manchester united is playing Chelsea. They can even predict who will win and at what margin. They know, thanks to the Cable network news, internet TV, Satellite TV etc, how many soldiers are killed in Iraq daily, and how many suicide bombings and how many people kidnapped by militants. They know the countries with the most relaxed immigration rules. But ask them, what is the health benefits of banana, or how does bush burning affect the productivity of the soil, or what a balanced diet is, and you will be surprised at their level of ignorance.

Our youths are acquiring information about other places and lands, while losing knowledge of their land, their environment, their culture and their people.

No nation can truly develop until it develops its deposit of local knowledge, preserve it and nurture it. True and lasting development is that which is home grown and not imported from other lands. Sustainable and affordable technology must be based on indigenous knowledge. The best solution to a nation's problem is that which comes from within, not from without.

In many indigenous societies, when a knowledge bearer dies his knowledge dies with him. Indeed, a lot of knowledge is being lost, knowledge that appears to be worthless mainly because it is not properly valued. There is a need to protect endangered knowledge as a world heritage. Today, we speak of protecting our environment from abuse, and also about protection for rare species of plants and animals. But equally important is the need to set up international efforts to protect and preserve indigenous knowledge. With every old person that dies in our villages, a whole library of books is being lost. We must therefore protect our indigenous knowledge, especially development knowledge. Africa has the least patented knowledge in the world, which reflects Africa's low level of development. The little that is patented is hardly exploited, due to un-enabling innovation and business environment. Patented knowledge creates rarity and value and encourages sustainable knowledge development.

Tacit knowledge is the unwritten and even unspoken knowledge that exist within a person or within a community. In local communities, people often know more than they can tell. This knowledge remains hidden to an outsider. The art of development is the ability to convert and exploit local knowledge to create relevant technology

A nation's ability to convert and exploit local knowledge is critical to its development. Sustainable development must be local before it becomes global. The idea of technology transfer could be deceptive. From our knowledge of history, there have been three ways of acquiring technology: it is either stolen or bought or locally developed. No nation transfers her technology to other countries free of charge.

### Functional knowledge

Functional knowledge refers to knowledge as an asset, skill, an advantage, a tool. It is not an end but a means. It refers to economic knowledge or know-how. It is knowledge of how to transform knowledge into goods and services. Functional Knowledge creates, adapts and uses knowledge effectively for its economic and social development. The most important thing for a nation is not its natural resources but its ability to create knowledge to transform its society and make available the basic necessities of life. Knowledge in this context is grossly neglected and unused in Africa. Most often, it is wasted. It has been observed that the most striking aspect of Africa is its wastefulness; its waste of knowledge. It is one major cause of underdevelopment in Africa and why Africa is the most backward continent in the world.

Knowledge is a process, a continuum, always evolving, becoming, flowing, emerging, and dynamic. It is always flowing. It cannot be monopolized, blocked, tied-down or controlled. Knowledge upgrades and renews cultures open to it and eliminates those closed to it. It has its own inner dynamism, flow and logic. It has its own way of spreading and is unpredictable. It is the force behind historical and social changes. As knowledge evolves, society changes, institutions change, people change; inferior knowledge [in terms of know-how and effectiveness] gives way to superior knowledge. Knowledge for development has a universal character even as it creates local identities.

Much of African culture is backward-looking and static and this is keeping over 70% of Africans in poverty. It lacks innovation and dynamism, and projects culture as a static, unchangeable way of life rather than an evolving and changing interaction of intelligent beings in society, thereby widening the gap between the African continent and the rest of the world. Many African universities and centers of learning harbor professors and 'scholars' who are not able to update their knowledge bases. They could only see the world as they were taught as students, and are not able to go outside their doctoral and master theses, and hold on to the same old ideas of 30, 40 years ago. Rigid and static knowledge leads to extinction.

Consider this: while there has been a rapid, breathtaking technological innovation in the field of medicine, there has not been a corresponding change in medical curriculum in Nigerian universities. That means that medical curriculum in Nigerian universities has undergone very minimal change in the past 30 years. A course in business administration, for example, is done the same way as it is done in, say, an American university, as if the student is an American. A law curriculum is arranged in such a way that pre-eminence is given to the study of laws that originated in Europe. The public administration curriculum in African universities was designed by European colonizers based on the colonial set-up they had in place to help them train Africans in managing the colonies. Ironically, the curriculum is still very much as it was handed over by the colonizers, with minimal change after over 40 years.

## Danger of fragmented knowledge

As it creates and renews, so can knowledge also destroy. Scientific, technical or ideological knowledge is often misused, misinterpreted or misapplied in such a way that it becomes a problem rather than a solution. Specialized or fragmented knowledge is often accused of being badly utilized and applied and can get out of control to the detriment of the society. It encourages unsustainable and self-centered ways of life. Just as absence of knowledge encourages undesirable poverty, specialized knowledge leads to mis-development and forces its way into application even if at the detriment of the existing culture. The discovery of uranium was good news to the modern world and the knowledge of uranium has led to nuclear technology. But it has led to the production of the first atomic bombs which were dropped on Hiroshima and Nagasaki in Japan. Since then, humanity is faced with the threat of extinction due to a proliferation of atomic bombs.

While the internet has opened up new frontiers of knowledge and encourages free flow of information globally, it has also imposed a pornographic culture on the world. Cable network television often exposed African youths to negative, consumerist influence. While agricultural development has led to availability of more food in the world and thereby reduces hunger, it has also encouraged genetically modified food which has grave health consequences, as evident in the alarming rise in incidences of cancer, heart, kidney diseases as well as viral diseases all over the world. While mobile telephones and wireless technology has turned the world into a global village and has improved communication and business interaction, it has also exposed us to dangerous radiations as well as immoral influences.

In Africa, what urgently needs to be taught is not just knowledge in itself but the love of knowledge and knowledge acquisition as a lasting concern. Most of African countries are not developing not only because they lack relevant modern development knowledge but also because they are inundated with irrelevant knowledge that keeps them from developing. Modern knowledge needs to be increased and anti-development mythological knowledge reduced. Rather than relying on foreign aids and foreign NGOs, Africa must take ownership of her future by improving her knowledge bases.

### A new world

It is amazing how obsessed the world has become with those nations that are striving to develop nuclear weapons. The fear is that such proliferation of weapons could lead to a third world war and put the future of the world in jeopardy. The fact, however, is that a third world war is already raging. It is a peculiar kind of war. According to Samuel Huntington, it is a clash of civilizations. The old world order is changing. The world is no longer made up of the west, understood as Europe and America, and the rest of the world. Today, new civilizations are emerging and challenging the old order, and insisting on their right to see things in their own way, and do things in their own way. The war is against imposition of a single viewpoint as the only valid one, against imposition of a single civilization as the model of civilization.

The greatest threat to human development and growth today is no longer the atomic bombs. The greatest threat is a mindset that compels us to believe that there is only one way of doing things, that there is only one form of civilization, that there is only one form of democracy or that capitalism is the only valid economic system. This mindset wants us to believe that only one species of plants is the good one; that only one form of medical system is valid, forgetting that people of different cultures had for centuries developed their own kind of medical system, which is equally valid. Cultural diversity, not monoculture, is the nature of life.

Thanks to the internet, there is so much knowledge now available to people of all races. But it is not enough to generate knowledge because there is so much irrelevant knowledge in the world. The big challenge is to know which knowledge is relevant. Knowledge is power only when it is relevant to the development of the nation. Science is only a Latin word for Knowledge. Knowledge is our destiny.

# CHAPTER FOUR

# PRINCIPLES OF HERBAL MEDICINE

## Re-educating our children about herbal medicine

Education is a matter of developing the whole person, not just a part of the person. To be educated is to be intellectually, morally, physically, psychologically, socially, spiritually as well as culturally balanced. It is possible to be intellectually learned but morally illiterate; or one can be an academic giant but culturally a dwarf.

## Herbalism

Herbalism is the art of collecting, conserving, utilizing and application of medicinal plants for the care and prevention of illnesses; and for the promotion of physical and spiritual wellbeing. The person who practices this art is called an herbalist. An herbalist is a man or a woman who has a broad knowledge of the medicinal uses of plants and uses the knowledge to help him/her and others. The trained herbalist can identify and differentiate one herb from the other. In African Communities, some plants are known to almost everybody as medicinal. For example, the Neem tree also called "dogoyaro" tree, is known generally to be good for the treatment of malaria. But the herbalist sees deeper than that and uses the same plant for many other medicinal purposes.

People often confuse the term herbalist with other terms such as native doctor, juju doctor, witch doctor, etc. In the minds of many Nigerians, there is no difference between the herbalist, native doctor, sorcerer, magician, diviner, witch or wizard. They are all the same. Thus, the term has 'pagan' connotation. The herbalist is often seen as a subject of fear, an "idol worshipper" who can kill at will.

### Our cultural traditions are not inferior

It is a fact that more and more people are turning to traditional medicine for help. It is common to see medical doctors advising their patients to go and try traditional medicine when they meet complicated cases. But on the general level, many Africans still associate traditional medicine with "paganism" or "juju". I know of many Christians who were compelled to try traditional medicine in their sickness. When they got better they became disturbed that they had gone contrary to their faith. The fact is that they got relieved after taking the traditional treatment, but their consciences inflicted a worse suffering on them. The Christian Church is not against the use of herbs for the promotion of good health. What the Church is against is such pagan actions as rituals, sacrifices, oath taking etc.

It is indeed very sad that many people die of simple sicknesses which can easily be cured by herbs that are growing around them. Africa is the most blessed of all continents when it comes to medicinal plants. It is said that of the 300,000 (three hundred thousand) species of medicinal plants growing all over the world, over 200,000 (two hundred thousand) are found in Africa. Yet

ANSELM ADODO, OSB

millions of Africans die daily of various sicknesses. Indeed, "my people are destroyed for lack of knowledge" (Hos.4:6).

Many Africans still have it somewhere at the back of their minds that their cultural traditions are inferior and primitive and should be de-emphasized. The more their buildings; their liturgy, music, dressing and even food appear Western, the more civilized they think they are. To be civilized then means to be able to think, eat, walk and speak like Europeans and Americans. Every African, whether he admits it or not, suffers from a deep-seated inferiority complex, and this is the cause of many of our problems.

### The problem of nomenclature

Part of the reason for this confusion is the fact that some Nigerian languages do not have separate words for the diviner, witch-doctor, wizard or sorcerer. In many African communities, one person can perform all these functions. However, these functions are not identical and should be properly distinguished. In Yoruba traditional religion we have the following religious persons who perform some major functions which are unique in their own ways.

1. *Diviners*:-These are those who deal with oracles. They get messages from the ORISA and foretell what may happen in the future. It is possible to have native priests who are also diviners, but not all diviners are priests. The diviner finds out from the ORISA the cause of certain problems and what can be done to solve them. Often he prescribes sacrifices to be offered. But it is the priest who is properly qualified to offer those sacrifices. The priest-diviner is combining

two major functions and he knows it. The diviner can offer minor sacrifices which really can be offered by anybody. But he or she cannot officiate in the temple. The diviner is called 'BABALAWO'.

2. *Herbalists*:-These are concerned with healing and caring for the sick with herbs. They are very knowledgeable when it comes to plants and their medicinal uses. There are priests who also are herbalists. But an herbalist is not necessarily a priest or a diviner. The herbalist is called ONISEGUN.

3. *Witch-doctors*:-These are those who specialize in witch-hunting and cure those who are bewitched. In contemporary parlance, we may call them exorcists. The witch-doctor is always a diviner because it is through the oracle that he detects who is a witch. But his divination is done with reference to detecting a witch. The witch-doctor is called *Atinga* or *Semio*. The *Atinga's* function is very highly specialized and demanding as well as dangerous. This is why they are relatively few.

### *Approaches to herbal medical practice*

According to a 1996 WHO report titled: <u>WHO Policy and Activities in the Field of Traditional Medicine</u>, there is a renewed, growing interest in herbal medicine all over the world. As there is a shortage of medical doctors and pharmaceutical products, most of the population in the developing countries still relies mainly on traditional practitioners (TMPs) including traditional birth attendants, herbalists and bonesetters, etc. The following figures are some examples of the ratio of the total Populations to medical doctors compared with traditional practitioners: in China, for example, the ratio of medical doctors to the total population is 1: 20, 000, compared with traditional practitioners to the total population Ratio of 1: 200; and in Swaziland, these figures are respectively 1: 10,000 and 1: 100. In Sudan, the ratio is about the same as in Swaziland. One third of the adults in America have used alternative treatment and about 60% of the public in the Netherlands and Belgium and 74% in UK are in favour of complementary medicine being available in the National Health system.

There are two approaches to herbal medicine practice, namely:

1. Clinic-oriented approach
2. Community-oriented approach

1. *Clinic—oriented approach*

> In clinic-oriented approach, emphasis is placed on scientific identification, conservation and use of medicinal plants. Laboratory researches and screening are done to determine the chemical composition and biological activities of plants. Great interest is shown in quality control of raw materials and finished products, and development of methods for large scale production of labeled herbal drugs.

> The herbal drugs are labeled and packaged in the same way as modern drugs. They are distributed through similar channels as modern drugs, that is, through

recognized health officials in hospitals and health centers. Huge sums of money is spent both by the government and non-governmental organizations to promote further researches on herbs. In this approach, there is hardly any interest in the socio-cultural use of the plants.

2. *Community-oriented approach*

The emphasis here is on the crude and local production of herbs used for common illnesses. Knowledge of the medicinal uses of herbs is spread to promote self-reliance. Information is given on how to prevent illnesses. This approach aims at applying simple but effective herbal remedies to common illnesses. The target is the local community. No interest is shown in mass production of drugs. The cultural context of the plants used is taken into account, and local perception of health and healing. Simple Herbal recipes are used for the treatment of such illnesses as cough, cold, catarrh, malaria, typhoid and ulcers.

### Finding a balance

The two approaches analyzed above are two extremes of the same reality. There is need to harmonize these two extremes to complement each other. There seem to be little cooperation between people working on both sides, though things seem to be improving gradually.

On the one hand, scientists, pharmacists and medical doctors who follow the clinic-oriented approach sneer at traditional health practitioners and look down on them. One the other hand, the Traditional healers guard their knowledge secretly and refuse to subject their activities to scientific research. One of the aims of this little book is to contribute towards bridging the gap between Traditional medicine and 'orthodox' medicine.

### What is the goal of medicine?

The goal of medicine is to prevent diseases. This may sound strange to our modern mind that tends to see medicine as WAR, a fight against viruses and illnesses. But in ancient times, right from the earliest philosophers and medical scientists such as Hippocrates and Imhotep, medical practice had aimed at disease prevention. And various methods are thought on how to prevent diseases. This is evident in the Chinese tradition of employing physicians to look after their emperor so as to keep him healthy. If for any reason the emperor falls sick, the salary of the physician is suspended until the emperor is back to good health. This emphasizes the fact that the work of the doctor is to prevent the patient from falling ill.

### Why do we fall sick?

We fall sick for three reasons:

1. When an unwanted external entity gets into the body.
2. When some needed nutrients are lacking in the body.
3. When our body immunity is weak.

Unwanted entities are bacteria, viruses and entities that get into our bodies from the air, water, food, soil etc and disturb the body's normal harmony. If we have the required amount of vitamins and other essential nutrients in the body, the body can easily take care of the unwanted external entities as soon as they enter into the body, otherwise, they will begin to cause damage in the body. The extent of the damage done depends on our defence mechanism.

## *What is a drug?*

A drug, broadly speaking, is any substance that, when absorbed into the body of a living organism, alters normal bodily function. A drug is a substance which has a marked/felt physiological effect. It is an energy whose effect can be felt. Note that the emphasis is on the effect, the kinetic. The substance itself is not defined. Therefore, any substance that is ingested with the intention of altering physiological action could be described as a drug. In pharmacology, a drug is "a chemical substance used in the treatment, cure, prevention, or diagnosis of disease or used to otherwise enhance physical or mental well-being."

## *What is a medicine?*

A medication or medicine is a drug taken to cure and/or ameliorate any symptoms of an illness or medical condition, or may be used as preventive medicine that has future benefits but does not treat any existing or pre-existing diseases or symptoms.

## *Energy is ability*

Energy is defined as the ability to do work. Cells convert potential energy, usually in the form of C-C covalent bonds or ATP molecules, into kinetic energy to accomplish cell division, growth, biosynthesis, and active transport, among other things. Energy exists in many forms, such as heat, light, chemical energy, and electrical energy.

## *What is thermodynamics?*

Thermodynamics is the study of energy.

### *Thermo-heat, dynamic-power*

The first Law of Thermodynamics states that energy can be changed from one form to another, but it cannot be created or destroyed. The total amount of energy and matter in the Universe remains constant, merely changing from one form to another. The quantity of matter/energy remains the same. It can change from solid to liquid to gas to plasma and back again, but the total amount of matter/energy in the universe remains constant.

The second Law of Thermodynamics is commonly known as the Law of Increased Entropy. While quantity remains the same (First Law), the quality of matter/ energy deteriorates gradually over time. This is because usable energy is inevitably used for productivity, growth and repair. In the process, usable energy is converted into *unusable* energy. Thus, usable energy is irretrievably lost in the form of *unusable* energy. In all energy exchanges, if no energy enters or leaves the system, the potential energy of the state will always be less than that of the initial state. This is also commonly referred to as entropy. A watch spring-driven watch will run until the potential energy in the spring is converted, and not again until energy is reapplied to the spring to rewind it. A car that has run out of fuel will not run again until you walk some distance to the station and refuel the car. Once the potential energy locked in carbohydrates is converted into kinetic energy (energy in use or motion), the organism will get no more until energy is input again. In the process of energy transfer, some energy will dissipate as heat.

### Kinetics

Chemicals may be considered from a potential energy or kinetic energy standpoint. One pound of sugar has a certain potential energy. If that pound of sugar is burned the energy is released all at once. The energy released is kinetic energy (heat). So much is released that organisms would burn up if all the energy was released at once. Organisms must release the energy a little bit at a time.

### Potential versus kinetic energy

Potential energy, as the name implies, is energy that has not yet been used, hence the term potential. Kinetic energy is energy in use (or motion). A tank of gasoline has a certain potential energy that is converted into kinetic energy by the engine. When the potential is used up, you're out of gas! Batteries, when new or recharged, have a certain potential. When placed into a tape recorder and played at loud volume, the potential in the batteries is transformed into kinetic energy to drive the speakers. When the potential energy is all used up, the batteries are dead. In the case of rechargeable batteries, their potential is re-elevated or restored.

### Energy of plants

All plants have potential energy. When this energy is used to treat an ailment, it becomes kinetic energy. Over 90% of plants energy exists as potential energy, because human beings are yet to discover their uses. Indeed, human search for knowledge is yet to begin, for knowledge is limitless.

### Pharmaco-kinesis is the study of how drugs work in the body

- Pharmakon-'drug', 'medicine'
- Kinetikos-'to move', 'to act'

A tablet of panadol has potential to relieve headaches. It has only a potential energy. When it is swallowed and it dissolves into the bloodstream, its energy becomes kinetic. Same energy, different mode. A bulb of garlic has potential to lower cholesterol level and improve metabolism. When it is eaten, its energy becomes kinetic. That means that the energy in the onion while remaining the same has moved from one state [potential] to the other [kinetic].

*Some criticisms of herbal medicines*:

1. Lack of standardization and of safety. This is said to be the biggest problem of herbal medicines.
2. It is technically difficult to identify with precision hundreds of chemical constituents that are in an herb.
3. Lack of scientific proof of its efficacy. The fact that a certain kind of treatment works is not enough, how it works is equally important.
4. Most of the claims of efficacy are not objective, as they are made by the practitioners themselves, and their diagnosis is often imprecise.
5. Most herbal medicines have no precise dosage.

In order to properly respond to these criticisms, it is important to consider the following points:

*Uses of herbs*

Herbs are used in three ways:

1. As Food
2. As supplement
3. As drug

Herbs, spices, condiments, fruits and vegetables are naturally occurring gifts of nature. They have been endowed with the unique capacity to absorb inorganic substances from the earth, water, fire, air, ether, and convert them into life-giving, life-supporting vital ingredients. The human body too is a living entity, and each individual body has its own life-force which sustains it. When we look for herbal remedies in natural substances, we want something we can easily assimilate.

The medicament present in these remedies is in the form of alkaloids, essential oils, enzymes, trace elements and minerals. Once absorbed they are assimilated only in the quantity needed by the body. The active ingredients are in the natural form needed to bind to a receptor site where the vital action takes place, in order to balance the disturbed agent. There are no synthetic constituents added, as in commercial preparations, which work on the principle that a vehicle (synthetic constituent) is needed to ensure the absorption of an arbitrarily decided, fixed amount of a drug.

The right natural herbal remedy, taken at the first physical symptoms, manifestations or signs of disorder, helps the body's own healing mechanism. Since these are alternative natural medicine and a part of one's daily diet, excess of any kind is excreted.

Bitter leaf, pawpaw, pumpkin, water melon and other fruits, vegetables and herbs are used daily by millions of people. As food, they are used to make soups, spices and other delicacies. The emphasis here is not just on their medicinal benefits but also their taste. For example, Bitter leaf soup [onugbu soup] a popular soup among the Igbo of eastern Nigeria, has almost become a national delicacy, available in many popular Nigerian eating joints. Before making use of bitter leaf for soup, the leaves are thoroughly squeezed to reduce the bitterness. But as a supplement, bitter leaves are squeezed in water and drunk, usually one glass in the morning and one glass in the night.

The same bitter leaf can be used as a drug. This involves a systematic extract of the active ingredients of bitter leaf following a set pattern of extraction to target some particular organs of the body, the pancreas for example.

### Criticism revisited

From the above discussion, it is clear that the criticisms leveled against herbal medicines are directed to their use as a drug. For example, the idea of precise dosage only applies when dealing with chemicals or synthesized plant extracts. In dealing with such substances, precise dosage is vital to avoid over dosing. But when herbs are used as food or as supplement, precise dosage does not really apply. The body simply takes the amount of nutrient it needs and the rest are excreted via the various body organs such as the kidneys and the skin. It is therefore wrong to impose a 'chemical mentality' on the use of herbs generally.

The issue of proper diagnosis is being resolved as more and more herbal practitioners employ the orthodox method of diagnosis before treatment. Also, there is now better cooperation between orthodox medical practitioners and herbal practitioners. Some herbal clinics now work hand-in-hand with orthodox practitioners who made diagnosis and then refer the patient to the herbal specialist for medication. In Nigeria, the PAX Herbal Clinic and Research Laboratories are pioneers in this approach to Medicare which is revolutionizing health care practice in Nigeria.

## Herbal medicine in Britain

The policy of the United Kingdom's government on herbal medicine is based on the "Doctrine of reasonable certainty. "This states that a substance's historical use is a valid way to document safety and efficacy in the absence of scientific evidence to the contrary.

## Herbal medicine in the United States of America

The policy of the American government is that herbal medicines can be labelled and sold as food supplements without any specific health claims. Clinical trials are mandatory before any official claim of cure can be made.

## What is 'cure'?

Cure refers to the elimination of pain that arose due to a deformity in the physical body. For example, an intestinal ulcer is a bodily condition whereby a wound occurs in the intestine. Treatment aims at eliminating the wound so that the patient no longer experiences the discomfort associated with intestinal ulcer. Malaria occurs when there is excess presence of malaria-causing parasites in the blood. Treatment consists in eradicating these parasites from the bloodstream. If and when this aim is achieved, a cure is said to have taken place. The same applies to all physical sicknesses. The aim is always to eradicate the sickness using the symptoms as guide. When the symptoms cease and the patient no longer experiences discomfort, and the corresponding diseased organ becomes normal, a cure is said to have taken place. In treating diabetes, the aim is to isolate the diseased organ, which are the pancreas; and administer them with some doses of the drugs. In hypertension, it is presumably the blood vessels that are defective. In cancer, it is the blood cells; in arthritis it is the joints and so on and so forth. When the diseased organ is brought back to a normal state, a cure is said to have occurred.

## The price of 'cure'

All drugs have side effects. Some drugs make you sleepy, others-like for example antidepressants-can give you a headache, while some, like Halfan, can make your heart beat fast. Why do drugs have side effects?

Our bodies are complex structures, built from chemicals and to function smoothly, it has to be regulated. Chemicals like for instance hormones, enzymes and other molecular messengers normally make these adjustments. The purpose of drugs is often to take the place of one of the body's regulating chemicals and do what should normally be done by the body's immune system. Our body often uses the same chemical to regulate more than one process. On the other hands, drugs are targeted at a particular organ. What this means is that a drug may repair not only the desired target but also others that don't need readjustment. Drugs are not always as selective as we would like them to be. A consequence of this is that the medicine may alter a number of unrelated processes at the same time. The antidepressant amitriptyline can help depression but it can also lower blood pressure by affecting norepinephrine receptors, cause blurred vision, dry mouth and constipation by blocking acetylcholine receptors and even induce sleepiness and weight gain by binding to histamine receptors.

Modern medicine laboratory or clinical drug trials, blind and double-blind studies, determine that a certain level of the drug has to be maintained in the body to rid it of nocuous symptoms. This by itself may initially have a beneficial effect, but sustaining pre-determined, 'scientifically' approved levels in the long run also gives rise to excess intake, drug-induced/drug dependent diseases.

### What is alternative medicine?

According to the world *encyclopaedia*, the term alternative medicine refers to any healing practice that does not fall within the realm of conventional medicine. In practice, alternative medicine encompasses therapies with a historical or cultural, rather than a scientific, basis. This definition is based on a western interpretation of alternative medicine.

### What is complementary medicine?

Complementary medicine is the term used to describe alternative medicine when used in conjunction with mainstream orthodox techniques.

### What is 'cam'?

In a 2005 report entitled *Complementary and Alternative Medicine in the United States,* the Institute of Medicine (IOM) adopted this definition: "Complementary and Alternative Medicine (CAM) is a broad domain of resources that encompasses health systems, modalities, and practices and their accompanying theories and beliefs, other than those intrinsic to the dominant health system of a particular society or culture in a given historical period. The National Centre (USA) for Complementary and Alternative Medicine (NCCAM) defines CAM as "a group of diverse medical and health care systems, practices, and products that are not currently part of conventional medicine."

David M. Eisenberg, Associate Professor of Medicine at Harvard Medical School, defines it as "medical interventions not taught widely at US medical schools or generally available at US Hospitals". Richard Dawkins, British biological theorist, defines it as a "set of practices which cannot be tested, refuse to be tested, or consistently fail tests."

The US Institute of Medicine [IOM] analyzed this approach to defining alternative medicine and found it problematic because some CAM is tested, and much of mainstream medicine lacks strong evidence. The IOM found that in a study of 160 systematic reviews of mainstream techniques, 20% were ineffective and 21% had insufficient evidence. Dr. Michael Dixon, the Director of the British National Health Service (NHS) Alliance stated that "People argue against complementary therapies on the basis of a lack of evidence. But I'd say only 10 per cent of what doctors do in primary care is evidence-based."

The IOM therefore defined alternative medicine broadly as the ***non-dominant approach*** in a given culture and historical period. Consequently, one may well conclude that since over

70% of Africans depend on it, Traditional Herbal Medicine is the conventional medicine or orthodox medicine in Africa, while western medicine is alternative or complementary.

## Evidence-based medicine

According to the National Center for Complementary and Alternative Medicine (NCCAM), formerly unproven remedies may be incorporated into conventional medicine if they are shown to be safe and effective. Several scientists share this point of view and state that once a treatment has been tested rigorously; it no longer matters whether it was considered alternative at the outset. If it is found to be reasonably safe and effective, it will be accepted. According to them it is possible for a method to change categories (proven vs. unproven) in either direction, based on increased knowledge of its effectiveness or lack thereof. Some scientists say that the claims made by alternative medicine practitioners are generally not accepted by the medical community because evidence-based assessment of safety and efficacy is either not available or has not been performed for many of these practices. If scientific investigation establishes the safety and effectiveness of an alternative medical practice, it may be adopted by conventional practitioners.

## Do herbs have side-effects?

When used as food and supplements, herbs have no side effects. However, as a drug, herbs can have from mild to severe side effects. This brings us to the second criticism of herbs: that it is technically difficult if not impossible to identify with precision hundreds of chemical constituents that are in an herb. It is a fact that fruits, vegetables and herbs contain hundreds of active constituents that are beneficial to health. When taken in their natural state, herbs benefit the body in various ways and different people can derive different benefits from the same herbs depending on their health needs. This explains why the same herb may be prescribed for different ailments. To the chemically-minded observer, this may sound 'unscientific'. What is needed is probably some degree of humility to acknowledge that the orthodox, conventional method of healing is not the only valid health system, and that there are other ways of attaining health that are equally valid.

### When to harvest herbs

Herbs [the leaves] should always be gathered fresh, before noon, when their natural oils are at the maximum. Herbal natural oils are highly volatile, and the steadily increasing heat of the ascending sun depletes them. The best time of season to harvest most herbs is just when the flower buds are forming, but just before they open.

### How to harvest herbs

Always use a sharp knife to harvest herbal stems, leaves and barks. Pulling at the plants with the fingers does damage to the root systems and will lead to poor growth patterns in the next season. Since you did not manufacture the plant, you have no right to maltreat or injure it. The plant deserves your respect and fair treatment. Remember that we humans are the youngest occupants of the planet earth. The plants and the animals were here before we came. Know what part of the plant you need. Some plants are used in their entirety, others only specific parts. When you are gathering plants from the wild, remember not to take all of a particular species you may find in an area. Leave some to grow and seed and flourish for the next time you need them. When taking leaves or branches of a plant, leave plenty for the plant to survive. Don't strip barks from around a tree trunk, as this will kill it. Instead, strip bark from small patches, or particular stems, to preserve the mother plant for later use, and to preserve its life. When using an entire plant, it is customary to hang the plant upside down in a dry area free from pests to allow the plant to dry. Make sure your herbs have dried thoroughly before storing them for further use, or you may discover that you have a moldy mess instead of a medicinal herb. Roots should be carefully washed, scraped, and chopped into small pieces to be sure they dry uniformly and thoroughly. Bulbs are tied together and strung up to dry.

### How to dry herbs

The greatest enemy of your harvested herbs is heat and light. Never dry herbs directly in the sun. Drying herbs in the sun exposes the volatile oils to sun rays and can make them lose up to 40% of their efficacy. Store your herbs in air-tight containers. The best containers to use are colored glass. The herb then does not pick up impurities from plastics, and does not eat through your plastics, as can happen. Store in a dry, cool area, and keep out of the light. This is the reason for using colored glass. Light can often break down the healing properties of your gathered herbs, shortening their shelf life and rendering them nearly useless after a short period of time. If stored properly, the shelf life of dried herbs is approximately one year. Tinctures can be stored for up to two years. Capsules should be used within one year. Once an herb has been ground, it shortens the amount of time the herb is effective. So do pay careful attention to when you have purchased or stored an herb, for maximum effectiveness.

### How to take herbs

### Take herbs before meals

As a general rule, it is better to take herbs on empty stomachs, an hour or two before meals. Taking herbs before meals is often convenient and the practice usually assures that herbs and foods are not mixed. However, taking herbs after meals may be necessary if the before meal dosing yields adverse gastric reactions.

### Do not mix food, herbs and drugs.

As much as possible, avoid taking food, herbs and drugs at the same time. Modern experience with drugs shows that simultaneous ingestion of a drug with a food or beverage can sometimes cause changes in absorption and effects. For example, ingestion of tetracycline with milk results in reduced absorption of the drug. People relying on protease inhibitor drugs (for HIV treatment) are well aware of the significant restrictions placed on the relationship of meals and drug dose timing because of lowered absorption when food is present. The general practice is to give an interval of 30 minutes to 1 hour between the ingestion of foods, drugs and herbs. Ingestion of certain pharmaceutical products with alcohol can cause adverse reactions because both produce a pharmacologic effect on the liver. It is possible that food components bind-up and therefore inhibit the absorption of various herb ingredients. The relatively low volume of herb materials consumed at one time (especially when not taking a high-dosage decoction) compared to the amount of food materials consumed suggests that it is possible for foods to inhibit the absorption of some herb components.

### Pregnancy and breastfeeding

While there are a number of herbs that can be very helpful for problems which arise during pregnancy, there are many more herbs which are NOT suitable for use during this time. We strongly advise that pregnant mothers do NOT take herbal remedies unless under the guidance of a qualified herbal practitioner. Herbs are absorbed into the bloodstream and are therefore likely to be present in breast milk. If you are *breastfeeding, please seek advice before using any herbal product.*

### Taking tinctures (liquid remedies)

Tinctures are a very handy way of taking herbs as they can be easily carried around in pockets or a handbag and taken in a small amount of water or fruit juice. The herbs are usually absorbed in about 15 minutes. The best time to take tinctures is between meals or up to 30 minutes before meals, unless otherwise advised.

## *Alcohol*

The alcohol content of 25-45% may be harmful to those suffering from alcoholism and should be taken into account in pregnant or breastfeeding women, children and high risk groups such as patients with liver disease or epilepsy. To reduce the alcohol content, add the required dose to a cup of freshly boiled water and allow to cool.

## *Dosage*

Guideline of doses for adults is given on each product label. Sensitive people or those of small stature may need to adjust the dose downwards. Try not to exceed the recommended dosage. Do not think that because it is an herbal product, the dosage does not count. Moderation is required in everything.

## *Infusion*

Infusion simply means "tea". Just like when you make tea, you pour boiling water over some leaves or flowers. That's what you do to make an infusion. A therapeutic dose will be one or teaspoons per cup, and let it stay for 10-15 minutes. Then you can add sweetener, juice or whatever you need as you desire.

## *Decoctions*

This is the most common traditional way to take herbs. It means boiling Herbs that look like roots and barks. Sometimes it takes hours to boil, and the smell and taste, which are often unpleasant, can hardly be controlled, no matter the amount of sugar or honey added.

# CHAPTER FIVE

# GIFTS FROM NATURE

***Psalm of Thanks***

*Thank you Lord*
*For what I am, for all I am*
*I thank you.*
*For my yesterday, my today and my tomorrow*
*I thank you.*
*For my father, mother, sister, brother, relatives and*
*friends I thank you.*
*For sun and moon and stars*
*I thank you.*
*For wind and water and fire*
*I thank you.*
*For earth and sky and mountains and valleys*
*I thank you.*
*For pawpaw and mango and banana*
*I thank you.*
*For rice and beans and cocoyam and cassava*
*I thank you.*
*For the grace to sing your praise daily*
*I thank you.*
*For what I am, for all I am, for what I will become*
*I thank you.*

## HEALTH BENEFITS OF BITTER LEAF

Everybody seems to know it. It grows everywhere. Bitter-leaf, (biological name *Vernonia amygdalina),* is a very homely plant. Wherever it grows, it flourishes an evergreen. The Igbo's call it Onugbu. The Yoruba's call it Ewuro. The Hausas call it Shivaka. Perhaps the most distinctive part of the bitter-leaf plant is its bitterness. Every part of the plant is bitter: the leaves, stems, root and bark. The Igbo of Eastern Nigeria use bitter-leaf mostly as a vegetable, while the Yoruba's use it more as medicine. Bitter-leaf is popular among old people for its bitterness. But the young people of today do not like the bitterness of the bitter-leaf. They would rather prefer biscuits, ice cream, chocolate and other sugary products. Their philosophy is "Life is sweet; therefore, food must be sweet."

The fact is that bitter herbs are good for the body. They remind us that life is not always sweet; that life is not a bed of roses; that both sweetness and bitterness are essential parts of life. Bitter herbs help to tone the vital organs of the body, especially the liver and kidney. The liver is the largest organ of the body. It weighs between 1-3kg in the adult. Its major functions are:

(a) Secretion of bile and (b) formation of glycogen. The liver is essential in the metabolism of fats and protein. Therefore it must be cared for properly. Once the liver has any defect, it is hard to correct. Every effort must be made to keep the liver in good condition. Alcohol, sugar and processed or refined foods can weaken the liver and make it susceptible to infections.

The kidney is another important organ in the body. The kidney is the organ that helps to expel waste materials from the body. It secretes urine that flows into the urethras. If the kidney breaks down, there is general disorder in the body. Bitter-leaf is very useful in the care of the kidney and the liver. This is the reason why we refer to bitter leaf as a cure-all. Because if the kidney and liver are healthy, the whole system will function well.

The bitter-leaf plant contains Vernodalin, Venomygdin and Saponin. Bitter-leaf should always be taken fresh. Boiling or cooking reduces the potency of most herbs. The Igbo of Eastern Nigeria eat a lot of bitter-leaf, but they often squeeze out the bitterness from the leaves before eating it. What is left then is mere chaff, with little or no medicinal value. Always remember that raw vegetables are better than cooked ones, and half-cooked vegetables are better than over cooked ones. Bitter-leaf, like other plants, is a sacred plant. Therefore, respect it and pray over the plant before you cut it. We need to cultivate an attitude of reverence for God's creatures so that we can be in harmony with them. The following are some uses of bitter-leaf.

1. *Stomach Ache*: Chew the tender stem of the plant like a chewing stick and swallow the bitterness. This is a well-known remedy for stomach ache. In some cases the ache stops within a few minutes. An alternative is to pound the fresh leaves in a mortar and press out the juice. Add a pinch of salt to three tablespoons of the undiluted juice and drink. This brings immediate relief.

2. *Skin Infection*: For skin infections such as ring worm, itching, rashes and eczema, the pure undiluted extract of

bitter leaf is excellent. Simply apply it to the affected area daily.

3. **Diabetes:** Diabetics should listen carefully to this good news. They do not need to despair or lose hope. God has not abandoned them. God has given them bitter-leaf as a sign of God's love and care. From time immemorial, herbalists have been using the bitter-leaf plant to treat diabetes. Bitter leaf not only reduces the sugar-level drastically, it also helps to repair the pancreas. Squeeze the juice from ten hands full of the fresh leaves in ten liters of water and take two glasses, three times daily for one month. This amounts to six glasses daily.

4. **Loss of Memory:** Loss of memory can be a symptom of diabetes, or a sickness on its own. Whatever its nature may be, bitter-leaf is good for this ailment. Take one glass three times daily for at least two months.

5. **Prostate Cancer:** Prostate cancer is common among men who are over forty years old. One of its symptoms is difficult and painful urination, among others. Bitter-leaf is very good for this ailment. It increases the flow of urine and reduces the pain, as well as regulates the spread of the cancer cells. Simply squeeze the fresh leaves in water and take a glassful four times daily. Don't be surprised if you begin to urinate very frequently after you take the bitter-leaf extract. It is part of the cleansing and healing process that your body needs.

6. **General Weakness:** Do you often feel weak and tired? Do you lack vitality and vigor? Then get up and take a walk into the bush. You don't need to walk far before you find

a bitter-leaf plant. Squeeze the leaves in water and take a glass three times daily. Once you follow this instruction, you will experience a new release of energy.

7. **Stroke**: Bitter-leaf solution calms the nerves, strengthens the muscles and cleanses the system. I have seen what marvels the bitter-leaf extract has done for many people and I can testify that it is good.

8. **Pneumonia**: Squeeze the fresh leaves of the plant in water. Take a glass-full three times daily. Warm the solution over a flame each time before drinking. Remember, do not boil (or use a microwave), just warm. Continue the remedy for a month. You do not need to squeeze the leaves each time you want to drink it. You can squeeze a large quantity once and add some honey. This will help preserve the solution. However, note that if you store bitter-leaf extract for twenty-four hours or more, the bitterness will disappear or diminish.

9. **Insomnia**: Bitter-leaf extract has done wonders for those suffering from sleeplessness. Simply take two glasses of bitter-leaf solution every night (you may add a little honey if you wish) and you will be calm and have great well-being.

10. **Arthritis**: Arthritis or rheumatoid patients who have tried bitter-leaf solution can attest to its effectiveness. It soothes inflamed joints and eradicates the pain.

## THE WONDERS OF PAWPAW

The pawpaw plant is a native of South America, where it was cultivated since Pre-Columbian times. There are 22 plants and trees in the pawpaw genus; the most famous of which is Pawpaw *(Carica papaya)* which reached Europe in 1690 and Asia in the 18th Century. Pawpaw is now grown all over tropical Africa. It is a very beautiful plant; hence it is used ornamentally in some parts of the world. Pawpaw is one of God's wonderful gifts to humanity. When one looks at the beauty and richness of nature, one cannot but burst into songs of praise to God. Pawpaw is a pharmacy in its own right. We all eat pawpaw and enjoy its sweet and pleasant taste. But how many of us know the medicinal values of this wonderful plant? Some time ago, I visited a poor old man living alone in a village house. His three children were working outside the country. The old man had an old sore on one of his legs that refused to heal despite regular medication. The sore was so bad that the man's leg was actually rotting away. "Why is no one treating you?" I asked him. He replied "My children all live abroad and they always send me Oyinbo (Western) medicine to cure my leg, but my leg is stubborn." My heart sank!!! At the back of this old man's house, were three healthy pawpaw plants. I drew his attention to the plants and showed him how to use the pawpaw fruit to treat his sore. Within three months his leg was healed and he was back to normal. He was able walk to the farm and to church. I did not have to bring Holy Communion to him at his home anymore.

How heart-wrenching it is to see people dying of common illnesses that can easily be cured. Go to our hospitals and you will see what I mean. Drugs are so expensive. The worst part is that seventy percent of the drugs in the Nigerian market are faked. What other hope do we have, but to turn to nature? I once spent the night with a simple family in a remote village, where I had gone to do research. After settling down, my host showed me to the bathroom and apologized that there was no special soap for me to bathe. I told him I did not need a special soap because there was natural soap growing nearby. I took him to the pawpaw plant in front of his house and showed him how to use the leaf as soap. The following morning he applied what I had taught him. He simply squeezed the leaves together and used them to scrub his body. He was excited at how effective it was. Such is the wonderful nature of the pawpaw plant.

Pawpaw improves the digestion of proteins and expels worms. The ripe fruit is rich in vitamin A, B and C. Vitamin A is good for eyesight, Vitamin B is good for the nerves and muscles, while vitamin C strengthens the immune system and helps fight against illnesses. To expel worms, chew two table spoons of the seeds of a ripe pawpaw fruit first thing in the morning and last thing at night. Do this for three days. Eat only fruits for breakfast and dinner for those three days. For chronic external ulcers or sores, cut a piece of unripe pawpaw fruit and apply it directly to the wound and secure it in place. Do this procedure four times daily. Continue for a few days or weeks until the wound dries. To make the wound heal faster, eat plenty of ripe pawpaw.

The following are some of the uses of pawpaw:

## Malaria Fever

Squeeze some yellow pawpaw leaves in water.

> **Dosage:** Take a glassful three times daily for seven days. The preparation is also good for jaundice and the dosage is the same.

## Diabetes

The green leaves of pawpaw are good for diabetes and for diabetes-induced hypertension. Squeeze the juice from the green leaves into a glass of water. Dosage: Take a glass three times daily. This is also good for constipation and the dosage is the same.

## Stomach Ulcer

Cut a big unripe pawpaw fruit into pieces. Do not remove the peel or seeds, simply cut the whole fruit into cubes. Then soak the cut fruit in five bottles of water for four days. Sieve the fruit from the liquid Dosage: Take half a glass three times daily for two weeks. This is a very good remedy for any type of intestinal ulcer.

## External Ulcer

The white milky sap of the unripe pawpaw contains a high percentage of papain, which is used for chronic wounds or ulcers. This can be obtained by making a slight cut in the skin of the unripe pawpaw fruit to allow the sap to drop. Papain is also present in the ripe pawpaw fruit.

## Convulsion

The dry brown pawpaw leaf is a good remedy for convulsion. Pick up the dry, fallen pawpaw leaves, clean them, and grind it into a powder. Add two tablespoons of the powder to half a glass of palm kennel oil (aka Palm Oil or Red Oil)

*Usage:* Stir well and rub the mixture all over the body. This preparation is really great for convulsion. It quickly arrests the abnormal condition and helps to bring down the body temperature when there is a high fever.

## Asthma

Burn dried pawpaw leaves

*Usage:* Inhale the smoke during an asthma attack. It brings quick relief. To prevent an asthma attack, inhale the smoke every night.

## Bronchitis

The root of the pawpaw plant is a good remedy for respiratory problems, especially bronchitis. Bring some pawpaw roots to boil.

*Dosage:* Take half a glass three times daily. For cough, simply chew a tender pawpaw root and swallow the juice.

**Piles:**    Pawpaw root is effective for the cure of piles.
Prepare the root the same way it is prepared for
bronchitis.

**Dosage:**    Take half a glass twice daily.

## Impotence

Cut two unripe pawpaw fruits into pieces (seeds and peel
inclusive). Bring to a boil in eight bottles of water.

**Dosage:**    Take half a glass three times a day.

## THE LIFE GIVING PROPERTIES OF WATER

Water is a life giver. Apart from air, there is nothing as essential
for life as water. The origin of water goes accounts of creation
in Genesis, we find that water is the oldest and most common
substance on earth. In the beginning, before creation, the earth was
a formless void; a mass pool of water covered the earth. Water is
also connected to the destruction of the world. When the Israelites
refused to obey God, God sent the flood to dissolve the world.
Water is then a principle of creation and dissolution. Note that I
say dissolution, not destruction, for God does not destroy. This is
indeed a mystery.

Right from the beginning, human beings have been fascinated
with water. Water is the strongest natural force in the world, far
more powerful than fire or wind. Everything on earth contains

water. We come from water and our survival depends on water. An apple is 80% water, tomato is 95% water, pawpaw is 90% water, and an orange is 95% water. The human body is 70% water and70% of the earth's surface is water. That is why water and water animals feature greatly in our dreams, we are water people. The symbolism of water is central to our Christian faith. In many places all over the world, people worship water. Water is the chief symbol of Christian initiation. At baptism we were immersed in water. It is important to note that immersion in water is not just a Christian practice; it is common to all religions. When an initiate is immersed in water, he/she is symbolically dead. Immersion in water symbolizes dissolution, end of the old life. When the initiate emerges from the water, he/she becomes a new person, with a new life. The old life is gone and everything is now new.

Even though water is the most common substance on earth, we actually use less than 10% of earth's water. Only 30% of earth's water is fresh water, and we use less than 10% of this. The rest exists as snow on the mountains and hills, and can't be used. Our earth is made up of hydrogen and oxygen. When hydrogen mixes with oxygen it becomes water. Water exists in three forms, solid (ice), liquid (water) and gas (vapor). Of all the natural substances on earth, water is the only one that exists in three forms. Water flows in oceans, rivers, and lakes. When temperature falls below 0°c, it changes to ice or snow. When temperature increases to 100°c, it changes to vapor or steam. To stay healthy, each person needs to drink at least 2 $\frac{1}{2}$ liters of water daily. A normal adult drinks between 60,000 and 70,000 liters of water in his/her life time. One can see that water is vital to healthy living. This is the reason why

I refer to water as medicinal. What we should learn, is how to avail ourselves of the life that water gives.

What are the functions of water? Let us state the obvious. The first function of water is to quench thirst, and the most natural thing for a person dying of thirst to demand for is water; not Coca-Cola, Fanta or beer. Water is the only substance that can really quench thirst. Processed liquid, such as soft drinks or beer only serve to suppress thirst for some time. They can never give you the same thirst quenching satisfaction that water gives.

Water aids the metabolism of food as well as washes the digestive system. It keeps the blood thin and light, so that it flows freely and smoothly, to supply the essential minerals needed for a healthy body. Water also moderates body heat, preventing it from rising too high or too low. Water serves as a lubricant for the muscles and joints, keeping them healthy and strong.

### *Water as Therapy*

Water therapy is a scientific method of drinking water to promote health and bring healing. When you wake up in the morning, drink at least five cups of water. It is better to do this as soon as you wake up, even before brushing your teeth. Drink more water during the course of the day; drink as much as you can, but never while eating. You should drink water at least one hour before or after meals, never during meals. This is because the body produces its own enzymes for digestion. So, drinking water while eating leads to a dilution of these enzymes, which makes the enzymes, lose their concentration. The safest and purest drinking water comes from springs. Before you go to bed at night, you should also drink two to three cups of water.

This is a simple method that can easily be taken for granted. However, its efficacy has been scientifically proven and documented. Cases of Diabetes, Cancer, Hypertension, Arthritis, Stroke and other illnesses have been reversed through water therapy. Let us make use of water for the health and betterment of ourselves, our children, and the world.

## THE MEDICINAL VALUE OF COCONUT

To many people, the Coconut plant is an ordinary plant. They do not see anything special or interesting in the plant. But to those who have eyes to see, the Coconut plant is a blessing, and a gift from nature. *Cocos nucifera* is called Coconut in English, Kwakwar in Hausa, Ivi-Obio in Edo, Ake-bake or Aku-oyibo in Igbo, and Agbon in Yoruba. It consists of glycerioles of capprylic, capric, lauric, myristic, palmitic, stearic, oleic and linoleic acids. Every part of this plant is medicinal.

The bark of the plant, when dried and burnt into ashes is an effective remedy for skin ailments like rashes, black spots, scabies and measles. Simply mix two-dessertspoons of the powder with half a glass of palm kernel oil. Apply to the affected area. For a toothache, mix two tablespoons of the ashes with one shot of dry gin. Stir it well and use as mouthwash.

### *Fibroids*

Cut the root into tiny pieces. Measure out fifteen handfuls of the pieces into ten bottles of water. Add 5 handful of *xylopia aethiopica*, called uda in lgbo, Erunje in Yoruba, and Unien in Esan. Bring to a boil. Then allow it to stand for 24 hours.

    ***Dosage:***    Take ½ a glass three times a day.

### *Bronchitis*

Chop an equal amount of pawpaw roots and coconut roots into pieces. Measure 10 handfuls of each into 10 liters of water. Add 5 bulbs of garlic. Bring to boil. Allow it to cool and add one bottle of honey.

    ***Dosage:***    Take ½ a glass three times daily.

### *Hepatitis*

Grind the dried coconut root into powder form and follow the formula below.

### <u>*Materials*</u>

- 8   dessertspoons of coconut root
- 8   dessertspoons of powdered bitter kola
- 2   tablespoons of powdered bird's pepper. Mix all together and add to 1 bottle of honey.

***Dosage:***    Take 2 dessertspoons three times daily.

This is a very effective remedy for hepatitis and jaundice. For dysentery, follow the prescription for Fibroids.

The water in the coconut is an excellent cleanser. It is among the best natural antibiotics known. Coconut water strengthens the immune system and helps to resist illnesses. If you are given some chemical antibiotics like Chloramphenicol or Amoxil in the hospital, you will or should be instructed not to drink coconut water because it will neutralize the effect of the drugs. If a child or an adult takes an overdose of a dangerous drug, you can administer coconut water to neutralize the side effects.

Four years ago, I met a lady who was diagnosed with breast cancer. It was so bad, that it was too late for an operation. I advised her to mix 4 liters of coconut water with 1 liter of honey and to take ½ a glass twice a day. The woman is still alive and going about her normal life even though the cancer symptoms are still very much apparent. The coconut water has a clearly moderate effect on the cancer cells. I am very sure that if an operation had been performed on the poor woman's breast, she would have died a long time ago. The white pulp of the immature coconut is very useful for our memory. People suffering from memory loss and any form of memory defect should make friends with coconut. Remove the whitish pulp inside the immature coconut and mix with a little bit of honey. Take as much as you wish. A trial will convince you.

## ALOE VERA—THE WONDER PLANT

Aloe is the name given to a variety of perennials of the Liliaceae/Aloeaceae family. There are over 325 species in this genus. *Aloe ferox*, *Aloe perryi*, *Aloe barteri*(West African Aloe), and *Aloe barbadensis* (*Aloe vera*) are the better known species. *Aloe vera* has been in much use from time immemorial. Wall paintings of ancient Egypt show that *Aloe vera* was used by the Egyptians to treat catarrh. Among the Jewish people, Aloe Vera was used as an ingredient for embalming.

The body of Jesus was wrapped with linen soaked in Myrrh and Aloes. Nicodemus brought a mixture of about seventy five pounds of Myrrh and Aloes. "Taking Jesus' body, the two of them wrapped it with the spices in strips of linen. This was in accordance with the Jewish burial customs." John 19:39-40. *Aloe vera*, a native of Southern and Northern Africa, came to Greece in the 4th century B.C., to China in the 10th century A.D. and finally, to Europe in the 11th century A.D. Even though there are many species, they all have similar constituents, namely: Antraquinone, Glycosides, Aloin, Resin, etc. Aloe Vera is the most common species of Aloes found in Nigeria today. This species grows well in flowerpots. It needs a balanced measure of sunshine and water to survive. It does not grow very tall (1-4 feet), and is light green in color with white spots. It is good to remember that there are many species of Aloes. One should not be surprised to see Aloes of different shapes, color or texture. The West African Aloe (*Aloe barteri*) has very broad succulent leaves and bright red flowers which can grow as high as 7 feet.

Since *Aloe vera* grows quickly, it should be planted in every compound. I have seen this plant growing in flowerpots in many compounds as an ornament. In some compounds, the plant is abandoned and starved for lack of water. Surely, *Aloe vera* deserves more honor and loving care. Below are some of the medicinal values of *Aloe vera,* the miracle plant.

## *Cancer*

A lot of research has been, and is being done on the efficacy of *Aloe vera* in curing cancer, especially breast cancer. I challenge our scientists to do more analysis of this wonderful plant. Rather than spending useful energy condemning and suppressing new ideas about health, let our medical health practitioners focus their attention on more intense research of medicinal plants that can save the lives of our people. Some time ago, I called one of my doctor friends, an "orthodox" doctor and told him I would like to discuss the issue of cancer with him. He said there was not much to discuss about, because cancer is incurable, and so I should not bother to discuss curing cancer with herbs.

Must our Nigerian "orthodox" doctors continue to fold their hands and expect their counterparts in Europe and America to do the thinking for them? In using *Aloe vera* for the treatment of cancer, one fact to keep in mind is that the older the plant, the more active it is. To treat cancer with the Aloe Vera plant, the plant must be at least five years old. The formula is as follows:

## *Materials*

3   Aloe Vera leaves
1   bottle of honey
2   bottles of dry gin

*Cut the leaves into pieces. Mix the bottle of honey with the 2 bottles of dry gin and grind it with the Aloe Vera leaves.*

**Dosage:**   Take 3 tablespoons twice a day for 2 months.

## Constipation

Constipation is a very dangerous ailment. It is a window for all other diseases. Constipation is the inability of the body to expel waste materials from the system. In constipation, metabolism is very slow leading to the decay of waste materials in the system. *Aloe vera* offers hope for those who suffer from this ailment.

To treat constipation, cut the root of an Aloe Vera plant into pieces. Soak one handful of the root in ½ a beer bottle of dry gin for one week. Then add water to fill the bottle. That will give you a full bottle.

**Dosage:**   Take one shot every night. This preparation should not be taken by pregnant women.

## Intestinal Ulcer

*Aloe vera* is one of the most effective remedies for ulcer that we know of. Since we have so much *Aloe vera* plant around us, it is sad to see so many people still suffering from ulcers. I remember a religious sister who came to me two years ago because she was suffering from a very stubborn peptic ulcer. She had gone to almost every hospital in Nigeria without finding a permanent solution to the problem. She was told eventually that her problem was psychological and psychosomatic. She consulted a number of psychologists, yet the problem persisted. When she came to me I prepared an *Aloe vera* mixture for her, the same way it is prepared for people with cancer.

**Dosage:**    Take two tablespoons three times a day.

By the third day, most of her symptoms had disappeared. She continued the medication for a month. Since then she has never experienced any of the symptoms. I hope more people will get to know about this wonder plant and avail themselves of the wonderful blessings of nature.

## Impotence

Impotence is one of those illnesses that is not spoken about publicly, but is very common. Whether we want to face it or not, impotence is a major factor in divorce among married couples today. Once again, Aloe Vera is there to offer hope and life.

Cut the root of *Aloe vera* into pieces. Remember that the older the plant the more potent it is. Soak two handfuls of the root in one beer bottle of dry gin for ten days. Endeavour to shake the bottle each of those ten days.

*Dosage:* Take six tablespoons two or three times daily, depending on your need. However, do not exceed six tablespoons three times daily.

## Suppressed Menstruation

*Aloe vera* is an effective remedy for all forms of gynecological problems, especially suppressed menstruation, anovulation and irregular menstruation. To treat these lists of problems, *Aloe vera* is prepared in the following manner:

## Materials

4   *Aloe vera* leaves
1   beer bottle of honey
½   beer bottle of water
4   tablespoons of dried powdered ginger

*Mix the honey and water and grind with the Aloe vera leaves. Then add the dried powdered ginger and mix.*

*Dosage:* Take 3 tablespoons three times daily for 1 month.

## Other Illnesses

The beauty of the *Aloe vera* plant is that it is useful for so many ailments. It is one of the most potent antibiotics in the world. Apart from the uses mentioned above, *Aloe vera* can also be used to cure illnesses such as liver and kidney problems, Piles, Eczema, Dandruff, Ringworm and Glaucoma.

It also has a modulating effect on the HIV virus. *Aloe vera*, the wonder plant grows near and around you. Cultivate this plant. Care for it and reap the abundant blessings which God has given to us through this plant.

## Herbal Cure for Diabetes

Diabetes is one of the most common diseases in our society today. It used to be regarded as the disease of the rich and affluent. But now, it affects even the poor, thanks to modern civilization and urbanization. But what is diabetes? It is a metabolic disorder caused either by a deficiency of the digestive hormone called insulin or the inability of body cells to use available insulin. When we talk about diabetes, there is one organ in the body that requires attention. The organ is called the pancreas.

## What is the Pancreas?

The pancreas is an organ that excretes the hormone insulin and pancreatic fluid which contains enzymes involved in the digestion of fats and proteins in the small intestine. The pancreas, which is shaped like a human tongue, lays below and behind the stomach and in-between the two kidneys. It weighs about 100 grams, and is made of small units called lobules. Each lobule consists of two groups of cells, the exocrine and the endocrine. The endocrine group of cells is called an "Islet of Langerhans". The beta cells of the Islets produce insulin while the alpha cell of the Islets produce glucagon, a hormone which does the reverse of what insulin does, that is, it causes a breakdown of glycogen into glucose, thus raising up the blood sugar level and preventing it from falling too low.

## Kinds of Diabetes

The term "Diabetes" as used in this book refers to "Diabetes Mellitus." There is another kind of diabetes called "Diabetes Insipidus" a condition of Polyuria (excessive production and/ or passage of urine) and Polydipsia (excessive thirst) due to a deficiency of Anti-Diuretic Hormone (ADH). This kind of diabetes is less common among Nigerians and so will not be considered. There are two types of Diabetes Mellitus; Juvenile Diabetes, also called Insulin Dependent Diabetes Mellitus (IDDM) and Maturity Onset Diabetes also called Non-Insulin Dependent Diabetes Mellitus (NIDDM). IDDM is common in children and young adults. The condition is characterized by a deficiency of Insulin in the body. Thanks to modern medicine, Insulin can be artificially injected into the body. NIDDM is common in middle-aged people. In this case, there is Insulin in the body, but the body cannot make use of the available Insulin.

## Causes of Diabetes

- *Heredity:* It is believed that heredity plays a part in the spread of diabetes. However, there is no explanation how exactly this happens. While it is true to say that diabetes tends to run in families, it does not necessarily imply that everyone born into such families will develop the disease. Nor does it imply that those who do not belong to such families will never get the disease. It is good to note that in families where diabetes tends to run, the members will have the tendency to get the disease, but if they take proper precautions, they may not develop the disease.

Some scholars have maintained that what is inherited is not the disease, but a lack of the chromosome that resists the disease.

- **Overweight**: It is said that 60 to 90 percent of diabetics are overweight. A high intake of carbohydrates and high calorie foods will lead to being overweight. This occurs when there is no balance between the intake of food and the digestion and utilization of the food. As a result extra calories are stored in the system. To cope with the extra calories, the liver, kidney and pancreas have to do extra work. Overworking these organs will eventually lead to a breakdown of these vital organs.

- **Lifestyle:** It has been said over and over again that our lifestyle is one of the major causes of diseases in general. But how many people are ready to listen? Even as food nourishes our lives, so can it also destroy our lives. When a mother feeds her child with soft drinks, sugar, ice-cream, biscuits, chocolate and other refined foods, she thinks she is doing the right thing. She thinks she is "civilized" and making her child "civilized," not knowing that she is destroying the life of her child. "When a man drinks expensive wines, eats excessive amounts of red meat, drinks beverages with plenty of sugar, he says to himself, "I am enjoying life," not knowing he is eating himself to death. It is therefore important to learn the art of proper food combinations if we want to stay healthy.

- **Wrong Medication:** Self-medication has become the order of the day. Hospital bills are hardly affordable, so people would rather go to Chemists and get whatever medications they think they need, than go and see a doctor.

The wrong use of medication as well as the long term use of some medications can damage the pancreas. Chemical drugs are dangerous and should be taken with caution. One should avoid them whenever possible. What use is Chloramphenicol if it cures Typhoid but destroys eyesight or hearing? Those who constantly take medications for asthma, arthritis, contraceptives, etc. are in danger of damaging their pancreas.

## Symptoms of Diabetes

If you do not have Diabetes, then be grateful, and be sure you do all you can to prevent it. For prevention, is better than cure. The symptoms of diabetes are many and varied. At the earlier stages, diabetes does not show any symptom.

In many cases, the disease is diagnosed accidentally when undergoing a check-up for other complaints. The following are some of the symptoms of diabetes:

> *Polyuria:* Excessive urination. This constant urination is the most common sign of diabetes, because of the high level of sugar present in the urea. If you find yourself urinating very frequently, check if your urine is sweet by tasting the urea. If it is sweet, be cautious. This may not be enough proof that you have diabetes, but it may be an indication and you should follow up with a lab test to confirm.

*Polyphagia:* Excessive hunger often experienced by diabetics. This abnormal hunger is only a reaction of the body to a lack of glucose, thus starving the body's cells. The patient is tempted to eat more and more. Yet, the more food is consumed, the more the glucose level rises and the more body weight increases.

*Polydipsia:* Excessive thirst due to the high quantity of fluids lost through urine. The body experiences dryness of mouth and excessive thirst and the diabetic has an intense craving for water but is never satisfied.

*Loss of Weight:* Because the cells are starved of glucose, the body begins to make use of stored fat to nourish the cells. When this continues for a prolonged period of time, the diabetic begins to lose weight.

*Weakness and Tiredness:* In addition to using body fat, the body also feeds on the protein in the body, leading to general weakness and tiredness.

*Itching:* Persistent itching all over the body, especially in the genital areas is a symptom of diabetes. This is true especially in women. If a woman persistently experiences itching in her genital area, a medical checkup is advisable.

## *Diet for Diabetics*

Food is medicine. Food is the most natural medicine on earth. One cannot talk about diabetes without talking about food, and about dietary habits. Food is a major factor in any illness. This is especially true in the case of diabetes. Any treatment of diabetes should begin with proper food combination. It is good to note that drugs do not cure any illness. Drugs only help to strengthen the immune system and aid the system in fighting against illnesses or help to alleviate the symptoms of illness.

So many people come to me and say, "Father, I have diabetes, please give me medicine to cure it." My first question is always, "What do you eat and how do you eat?" The answer is nearly always the same, "My doctor told me to eat plenty of meat, beans, plantain and avoid yams, cassava, honey, fruits and sugar." "How many times do you eat in a day?" The response is typically, "At times twice a day and other times, three times a day."

As a diabetic, it is not good to eat only twice or three times daily, for such meals are often heavy. If a heavy meal is eaten even once a day, the body's sugar level will rise because there is insufficient insulin in the body to metabolize the large quantity of food. The key is to eat small portions of food throughout the day. For example, eat five or six times daily, but just a little at a time. Failure to observe this simple rule has sent many diabetics to the grave. In spite of all the complicated and expensive medications, they did not get better.

Food consists of carbohydrates, proteins, fats, vitamins and minerals. To be healthy, we need to maintain a balance of these nutrients in our diet. Carbohydrates include sugar, starch, cassava, yam, rice, etc. Protein is found in meat, fish, eggs, milk, beans etc. Saturated fats are found in butter, coconut oil, palm oil, meat and eggs. This kind of fat is dangerous for the system and can lead to heart disease. Unsaturated fats, which are derived from groundnut oil, soya bean oil, olive oil, cotton seed oil, castor oil, and various nuts (peanuts, almonds, etc.) are much healthier.

Vitamins and minerals mainly come from fruits and vegetables. Keep in mind that fruits and vegetables are best when eaten in their natural state. Raw vegetables are more nourishing than cooked ones. So often, I hear diabetics say that they have been told to abstain from eating fruits like pawpaw, bananas and oranges, as well as natural nectars like honey. But honey is good for the body. What is not good for the body is diluted or mixed honey. The sugar in honey is pre-digested and cannot be compared to the artificial, refined honey sold in the market. The sugar content of natural honey is only 7%, even though it is sweet. If diabetics do not eat fruits, how can they survive? What is bad is not the fruits, but the manner in which we eat it. Do not combine fruits with any other foods. This is a mistake which so many diabetics make. If you want to eat pawpaw, eat only pawpaw and not in combination with rice, beans or any other food. If you want to eat banana, eat a little at a time and do not combine it with any other food. If you want to eat green vegetables, please do, but do not combine it with Pawpaw. The key is to eat a little at a time. Eat plenty of onions, carrots, garlic and ginger. Eat green vegetables in their natural state as much as possible. Green leaves such as bitter leaf and pawpaw leaves are very good for the body. So often, people squeeze out the bitterness from the bitter leaves before cooking, thereby rendering the leaves useless. The bitterness is what actually makes the bitter leaf medicinal. Okra is very good for diabetics. Learn to eat your plantain or beans with okra soup.

## *Herbal Treatment for Diabetes*

To treat diabetes with herbs, the focus is to:

- Repair the pancreas
- Strengthen the kidneys
- Eradicate symptoms
- Prevent sugar or glucose from escaping in the urine
- Help the body to find its natural balance

## *Points to Note*

The following points should be kept in mind when treating diabetes with herbs:

- Juvenile Diabetes or Insulin Dependent Diabetes are more difficult to cure than Non-insulin Dependent Diabetes.
- Those who develop maturity onset diabetes at age fifty and above respond more quickly to herbal treatment than those who develop the disease at the age of thirty or forty.
- Insulin-dependent diabetics are not recommended to stop injecting themselves as soon as they begin herbal treatment. They will need to combine both medications for two weeks after which they will reduce the volume of insulin they inject to half the usual volume while they continue with the herbs. After four weeks, that they can put the insulin injection away, but only on the condition that they check their urine and blood sugar levels from time to time. That way they are able to monitor their sugar levels. Please make sure you consult a competent herbal scientist.

*Formula 1*
*Materials*

Cashew Stembark (half small bucket)

7 Green Pawpaw Leaves
1 medium size pot of Bitter Leaves
10 bulbs of garlic
10 fingers or pieces of ginger
5 bulbs of Onions
10 pods of *Capsicum frutescence* [English-African Red Pepper or Bird's Pepper (the smallest pepper you find in the market and is very hot). In Igbo—Ose Olibo, in Yoruba—Ata Eiye, in Hausa—Barkono, and in Esan—Usira].
15 pieces of Xylopia *aethiopica* (in Igbo—Uda, in Yoruba—Erunje, in Hausa—Kimba, and in Esan—Unien).
15 liters of water
2 bottles of honey

Boil all the materials together in pot containing 15 liters of water for minutes. Allow it to stand for 24 hours before adding the honey. Stir well and sieve, then store in a container.

*Dosage:* Take one glass 3 times daily for two months.

*Formula 2*
*Materials*

Leaves of *Mormodica charantia*(In English; Balsam Pear, In Yoruba: Ejirin)

Leaves of *Basil ocinum*(In Yoruba, Efirin, In Igbo, Nchanwu)

10 liters of water.

*Squeeze an equal amount of the leaves of the Balsam Pear and Basil leaves together in the water. Do not worry about the precise quantity of leaves. What matters is to squeeze equal amounts of both leaves and to make the preparation as thick and concentrated as possible.*

**Dosage:**    Take1 glass 3 times daily for 2 months.

## Arthritis is Curable with Herbs!

Arthritis is a disorder of the joints. The term "arthritis" comes from two Greek words, "Arthon" which means joint and "itis," which means inflammation. Arthritis therefore, refers to the inflammation of joints. There are over one hundred types of joint disorders, even though, they are all related. They are characterized by pain, swelling and stiffness, and at times, deformity. Rheumatism is another word often used in place of arthritis. Its meaning is rather vague and means different things to different people. In Nigeria the term is used for various aches and pains in the muscles and joints as well as for pains in general.

What is a Joint? A joint is where two bones meet. There are two categories of joints, immobile and mobile joints. Immobile joints refer to the inflexible and semi-flexible joints of the body. These joints do not move much as they have no cavity. An example is the head and spinal cord. Mobile joints are the flexible joints of the body. Examples are, the shoulder, knee, waist, toe, fingers, etc. They all have a cavity. These joints are technically called Diarthrosis (the ability of some joints of the body to move in several directions).

## Types of Arthritis

There are two main types of arthritis, namely Osteoarthritis and Rheumatoid Arthritis. Osteoarthritis is the most common type of arthritis. It is the degeneration or wearing out of a joint due to old age, over-exertion, or injury. Osteoarthritis affects the mobile joints of the body. Rheumatoid Arthritis is an inflammation of the same joints on the two sides of the body. For example, pain that is experienced in the right knee or shoulder is also experienced on the left knee or shoulder. The symptoms tend to come and go. Rheumatoid arthritis is very common in these days of processed and artificial food and drinks. It affects both the young and old, even infants. It is more common between the ages of 25 and 55.

## Causes of Osteoarthritis

There are two kinds of osteoarthritis; primary and secondary. Primary osteoarthritis occurs when joint degeneration sets in without any abnormal or apparent cause, while secondary osteoarthritis is that which has a known cause. The causes can be any or all of the following:

- *Heredity:* Osteoarthritis can be hereditary when parents pass it on or are disposed to a certain degeneration of the joint.

- *Excessive Stress:* If a joint is dislocated or injured and yet is still being exerted, arthritis may occur.
- *Previous Damage:* Untreated dislocation or half treated fracture will eventually lead to arthritis. Athletes who engage in physical exertion are often tempted to manage a dislocation or fracture. The eventual result is arthritis.
- *Overweight:* Accumulation of excess calories add more weight to the body. Extra body weight puts too much stress on the hips and knees. This results in arthritis.
- *Occupation*: One's occupation plays a major role not only in the development of arthritis but in the quality of one's health in general. Those who stand for long hours every day are prone to pain in the knees. Those whose occupation requires lifting heavy objects are also prone to waist pain, technically called lumbago.

### Causes of Rheumatoid Arthritis

There is no uniform agreement about the causes of rheutoid arthritis. Below are some of the possible causes, over and above the ones already mentioned.

- *Viruses:* Some scientists have proposed that rheumatoid arthritis can be caused by some kind of infection caused by viruses, leading to an inflammation of joints. These viruses are peculiar and live in the body for a long time undetected before their influence is felt.
- *Immuno-deficiency Syndrome:* This refers to a condition whereby the anti-bodies that are meant to fight against

foreign agents in the body begin to attack the tissues of the joints causing inflammation and pain.

## Symptoms of Arthritis

Rheumatoid arthritis usually begins with pain and stiffness in one or two joints, mostly the hands and feet. Initially the pain comes and goes. It is often worse when one wakes up in the morning, but wears off as the day progresses. Gradually, the pain becomes intense with constant swelling and inflammation in the joints. Moving or touching the joints becomes painful. The arthritis may soon spread to other parts of the body such as the elbows, knees, hips, waist, ankles, shoulders and neck. The person affected feels generally weak, tired, feverish and pale. The eyes become dry due to a reduction of tears. The mouth also becomes dry due to a reduction of salivary fluid, leading to a lack of appetite, followed by weight loss.

## Managing Arthritis

To treat arthritis, the focus is:
To strengthen the bones.
To repair damaged joint tissues.
To strengthen the weak joint tissues.
To strengthen the immune system against bacteria and viruses.
To eradicate the symptoms.
To achieve these results, diet plays a big role and is very important. Processed or refined food and drinks like biscuits and ice-cream and foods high in sugar must be avoided. Stop smoking, drinking coffee, and alcohol of all kinds must be avoided. Drink plenty of

water, especially first thing in the morning when you wake up. Try to eat just fruits for breakfast with water as your drink.

*Formula 1*
*Materials*

1   bottle of lime juice
1   bottle of grape juice
1   bottle of honey
Mix all together

**Dosage:**   Take 1 shot three times daily for two weeks.

**Side Effects:**   This formula may cause intestinal pain in ulcer patients, and should therefore not be taken by patients with ulcers.

*Formula 2*
*Materials*

8   handfuls Eucalyptus leaves
8   handfuls green pawpaw leaves
8   handfuls umbrella or fruits leaves
8   handful bitter-leaf
10  bottles of water

Boil all the materials together in a pot.

**Dosage:**   Take 1 full glass three times daily for one month.

*Formula 3*

**Materials**

6   handfuls pineapple peel

6   handfuls lemon peel

6   handfuls peel of unripe pawpaw.

10  bottles of water

Boil all the materials together in a pot.

**Dosage:**   Take 1 glass three times daily.

# LEMON—THE TREE OF LIFE

Citrus is a genus (set of closely related species) comprising of some 16 species of trees. The more known species are Lime, Lemon, Orange, Grape and Tangerine. Lemon is called the tree of life because of its many medicinal properties. The leaf is rich in aromatic essence, limonene and linalool. The rind contains 0.5% essential oil, which consists of limonene, coumarin and flavonoids. The juice contains Vitamin Bl, B2, and C; flavonoids and organic acids. A lot of research has been done on this plant. Its medicinal properties are scientifically proven and recognized. This is one of the contributions modern science can make to help promote traditional medicine. Rather than dismiss the claims of traditional medicine, science should use its complex technical apparatus to clinically verify these claims. Below are some of the medical uses of Lemon. Please note that whatever is said of Lemon, here is also true of the other citrus species, though to a lesser degree.

*Leaf:* Lemon leaf is a sedative and an antispasmodic (controlling spasms). For insomnia, nervousness and palpitation, soak 5 to 7 leaves of lemon in a teacup of hot water and allow it to infuse for 15 minutes.

*Dosage:* 1 cup two times daily.

Lemon leaf will serve as a good and better alternative to Valium and other synthetic sedatives, which have adverse side effects. To get the maximum results from Lemon leaf, take the preparation daily for at least one month. Do not expect that your insomnia or nervousness will disappear overnight. For migraine headaches and asthma, soak 2 handfuls of fresh Lemon leaves in a bottle of hot water and allow to infuse for 10 minutes. This should be taken warm. This applies particularly to asthma patients.

*Dosage:* Drink 2 cups every night for two weeks.

Lemon leaf is also good for worms. To treat worms, prepare it the same way it is done for migraine and asthma above.

*Dosage:* Take 3 cups every night for one week.

Fruit Rind: Lemon rind is a good remedy for lack of appetite, indigestion, constipation and typhoid fever. Add the rind of 10 Lemons to 4 liters of water and bring to boil.

*Dosage:* Take 1 cup 3 times daily.

Like the leaf, Lemon rind is a good worm expellant.

*Juice:* Lemon juice is an excellent remedy for scurvy, a disease caused by lack of vitamin C. Vitamin C (ascorbic acid) is found in fruits and vegetables. Hence, scurvy is common among those whose diet is poor in fruits and vegetables. Drink half a glass of Lemon juice twice daily. You may sweeten it with honey if you wish. For indigestion, mix half a glass of Lemon juice with half a glass of water and drink daily. This stimulates the activity of the digestive organs and strengthens the system. Due to the presence of hesperidins (chemical compound from citrus fruits), diosmine and other flavonoids, Lemon juice and rind improves blood circulation and so are good for Oedema, hemorrhoids, heart problems, stroke and hypertension. It is scientifically proven that Lemon produces alkalinization of the system, thus cleansing and re-invigorating the system. For tonsillitis and sore throat, mix half a cup of Lemon juice with four dessertspoons of honey. Warm it on the fire and use it to gaggle every morning and night. Lemon juice is very good for washing wounds. Steep a piece of cotton wool in the raw juice and use to clean the wound. Remember that Lemon juice is best taken fresh. It is not advisable to store Lemon juice for a long time. A lot of people have developed a habit of taking vitamin tablets daily. What those people need to know is that fruits and vegetables are the best source of vitamins there are. Lemon is a good source of vitamins. Lemon juice is very good for kidney stones.

Citrates [Citric acid salts], which are present in Lemon, not only prevent formation of kidney stones, but also help dissolve them. Drink half a cup of lemon juice two times daily. You may dilute it with water or sweeten it with honey, depending on your taste. An alternative way is to dry Lemon seeds and then grind into powder. Then Mix one teaspoon of the powder with two dessertspoons of honey, then lick daily for three weeks. Never mistake the so-called bitter Lemon soft drink for real Lemon juice, far from it! In fact, it is not good for the body as it contains carbonic gas and sugar.

To treat arthritis, kidney stones, gout, constipation and hypertension, there is nothing as effective as the famous Lemon therapy. Lemon therapy is capable of rejuvenating the body system and clearing the body of all toxins and waste product, giving a feeling of well being and lightness. Lemon therapy is indispensable in the treatment of cancer. Lemon therapy involves drinking the juice of Lemon in the following way. Take one Lemon the first day, then Increase it to two the next day. Continue to add one extra Lemon each day until the tenth day. Then begin to take them in the reverse order, subtracting one Lemon each day. If you wish to apply Lemon therapy please be sure to follow strictly the procedure above. It is one of the natural therapies that have been scientifically proven to be curative. It is very important to apply the therapy as described above. Ulcer patients should not apply Lemon therapy, as it may aggravate their condition. During Lemon therapy one should drink as much water as possible and eat plenty of fruits and vegetables. Solid food should be taken only once a day. Considering the abovementioned medical values of Lemon, you would agree with me that Lemon is indeed a tree of life.

# MISTLETOE:
## NATURE'S POTENT CURE ALL

Mistletoe, the parasitic plant, is a peculiar plant. Its roots sink into the branches and trunks of other trees, instead of into the soil. The seeds need sunlight to germinate, unlike most other plants that need darkness. The leaves produce chlorophyll even in the darkness, unlike other plants that turn yellowish when there is no light. The Mistletoe is an evergreen plant that does not die easily. As a parasite, mistletoe is a disease on other plants, which makes farmers to dread the plant. Mistletoe produces toxic berries, which are eaten by birds that spread them to other trees. Being gelatinous, the seeds stick easily to the trees and so they germinate there, Mistletoe, *Viscum album*, belongs to the Lorantaceace family of plants. The leaves contain choline and acetylcholine, which act directly on the autonomic nervous system. The berries contain alkaloids and toxic substances. For this reason we advise against any form of internal application of the berries.

### *How to Preserve Mistletoe*

Collect fresh leaves from the tree. The best time to collect mistletoe in a tropical country like Nigeria is between 12 noon and 1pm. As soon as you collect the leaves, rinse them in water, and then spread them out on a mat or zinc in an airy place. Do not expose the leaves to direct sunlight for more than one day. This is generally true of all herbs. It is always better to dry fresh leaves in a shady but airy place. It takes seven to ten days for mistletoe leaves to be properly dried. As the leaves dry up they tend to turn dark in color. Indeed, the mistletoe is a very peculiar plant.

## Kinds of Mistletoe

The mistletoe on Guava, Kola nut, Cocoa and trees of the citrus family are the most potent kinds of mistletoe. All others are also good but may not be as effective as the ones mentioned above. For the treatment of Cancer, the mistletoe on Guava is the best. This is because it contains the highest concentration of lectins, a kind of protein that science has discovered to destroy cancerous tumors and cells. It is the mistletoe on Guava that actually cures cancer. This important piece of information is known to some herbalists who keep it close to their chest. I am giving this information here, so that humanity may profit from it. To treat cancer, I recommend the mistletoe on Guava trees. To treat hypertension, nervousness and insomnia, I recommend the mistletoe on kola nut and the citrus trees. The mistletoe on cocoa is best for diabetes. However, these are observations based on practical experience rather than on purely academic scientific research, unlike in the case of Guava. I invite our scientists to verify these observations. For all other forms of illnesses, mistletoe on any edible fruit would help.

### *Methods Of Preparing Mistletoe*

### *Method One: Infusion*

Soak three dessertspoons of dried and powdered leaves into a cup of hot water. Allow it to infuse for fourteen to fifteen minutes before drinking. You may add honey if you wish. Do this two times daily.

### *Method Two: Cold Extract*

Soak two handfuls of the fresh or dried leaves in one cup of cold water for eight hours or simply overnight. On the following day add one cup of hot water to it. Sieve and store in a flask. Drink one cup in the morning and one cup at night. Mistletoe is well known for treating the following diseases:

### *Hypertension*

Mistletoe not only lowers blood sugar but also helps to repair the pancreas and other diseased organs in the body. Mistletoe is one of the most effective, if not really the most potent herb for hypertension. No matter how serious or chronic the case may be, mistletoe always makes a difference. Follow method one or two as described above.

### *Heart Problems*

Mistletoe is an excellent herb for the circulatory system. It promotes the flow of blood to the brain and heart, especially in those suffering from coronary artery disease and angina pectoris. Mistletoe is the safest herb for heart problems. In treating patients who have heart problems, great care must be taken to take the correct herbs or drugs, since any minor mistake could be fatal. When using mistletoe, there is nothing to be afraid of, because its efficacy has been proved and confirmed. Follow method one or two as described above for three months.

## Insomnia

Mistletoe relaxes muscles, calms the nerves, and eases palpitations, migraine, nervousness and pains. Those who suffer from epilepsy will find mistletoe very helpful as it protects against attacks.

## Arthritis

Mistletoe increases the production of urine and the elimination of toxic wastes from the system. Those who suffer from arthritis, rheumatism and gout have testified to the efficacy of mistletoe. Where other herbs have failed, mistletoe has proved to be a savior. External application of mistletoe is recommended in cases of arthritis, rheumatism and gout. Soak three handfuls of dried or fresh leaves in one bottle of water for two days. Deep a napkin in the solution and place it on the painful, swollen or inflamed joints. This brings a quick relieve.

## Infertility

For different forms of fertility problems, mistletoe has proved highly effective. Drinking two cups of mistletoe daily will correct gynecological problems, such as excessive menstruation, painful menstruation, irregular menstruation, anovulation, Amenorrhea and uterine hemorrhage. For Fibroids, drink three cups of mistletoe daily for six months. I recommend the mistletoe on Guava for Fibroids. I know a lot of women who faithfully took this medication and were patient enough to complete the six-month mistletoe therapy. Today they are not only free of fibroids, but are enjoying a new ease of life, for mistletoe rejuvenates.

## Cancer

Herbalists have been using mistletoe to treat cancer long before modern science did any research on it. Breast cancer is the most common type of cancer in Nigeria. Many women have fallen victims to this ailment. Radiotherapy, chemotherapy or breast excisionare temporal remedies; they do not cure the sickness. Mistletoe offers hope to all cancer patients. However, managing cancer with mistletoe is a long term affair. We must get rid of our modern day mentality that wants immediate solution to every problem. Recovery is a slow process. Herbs work slowly but more steadily and surely. For the treatment of cancer, soak three handfuls of dried mistletoe leaves in one beer bottle of water overnight. Then on the following day, add half a bottle of hot water. This will give one and a half bottles of solution. Drink one glass four times daily. Even though you will start to feel healthy within two months, you have to continue this treatment for six months. Don't get carried away. Follow the given prescription.

## Diabetes

I do not want to go into the issue of whether diabetes is curable or not. That is no longer an important issue. The most important question today is; what is the most effective plant for treating diabetes? I stand to affirm that mistletoe is among the most effective herb to treat diabetes. I know many diabetics that have never taken western drugs for the past five years, because they depend solely on mistletoe. Many of them simply drink a cup of mistletoe solution once a week. In the more serious cases of diabetes, I recommend the same dose that is given for cancer above, for six weeks. After that follow either method one or two of preparation and continue for five months.

## *General Health*

Mistletoe is not meant for the sick alone, it is also recommended for those who wish to remain healthy. Drinking a cup mistletoe tea daily will ensure protection against diabetes, malaria, typhoid, migraine, hypertension, pneumonia and all other physical ailments. As anti-malaria, we are yet to discover herbs that are as effective as mistletoe. For general health, drink two cups daily. I prescribed this for a middle-aged man two years ago, who used to suffer from serious attacks of malaria fever every two weeks. Even though he went to the best hospitals around and was given the latest malaria drugs in the market, it was to no avail. The fever kept coming every two weeks. It got to a stage that all the medical doctors treating him became frustrated and said to him: we are tired of you. Until this moment, this man has stopped suffering from malaria fever attacks. Mistletoe is indispensable for those suffering from HIV/AIDS. I always marvel at the efficacy of mistletoe for treating HIV/AIDS.

Within a month of mistletoe therapy, one would notice that almost all the symptoms such as fever, weakness, dysentery, and weight loss have been arrested. Now the patient can go back to work. I believe that mistletoe is one of the keys to unraveling the HIV/AIDS menace.

# THE HEALING POWERS OF GARLIC

Garlic, *Alliums sativum,* belongs to the Alliums family, which comprises of 700 species. Garlic is among the earliest known medicinal plants. The Babylonians [c.3000 BC] are said to make profuse use of garlic. The Jews love garlic and when they were deprived of garlic in the wilderness, they grumbled. *The rabble with them began to crave other food and again the Israelites started wailing and said, "if only we had meat to it! We remember the fish we ate in Egypt at no cost, also cucumbers, melons, leeks, onions and garlic. But now we have lost our appetite: we never see anything but this manna!"* [Num 11: 4-6] Garlic would surely restore their loss of appetite. Garlic was widely consumed in ancient Greek and Rome. Aristotle recommended garlic for those who wish to remain strong and healthy. The Roman soldiers were found to remain strong and healthy. The Roman soldiers were found of planting garlic in vegetable pots near their abode" since they believed that eating garlic would improve their fighting spirit.

The father of modern medicine, Hippocrates prescribed raw garlic for bronchitis. The tomb of the Egyptian king, Tutankhmen was said to contain six bulbs of garlic, to ward off dangers on his way to the other world. There are many myths and legends about garlic. One Muslim legend said, when Satan left the Garden of Eden after the fall, garlic sprang up from his left footstep and onion from the right.

In the 17th century in Europe, garlic was believed to ward off vampires and make moles to jump out of the ground. Greek athletes were given garlic to chew before competitions in Olympic games to help them run faster or excel. In ancient Greek, those who smelt like garlic were not allowed to enter the temple of Greek gods.

In the middle ages, physicians used masks mashed with garlic when treating patients with infectious diseases. In Ayurvedic medicine, garlic is called rashona, meaning, "lacking one taste". This refers to the fact that garlic possess all the other five tastes. They are pungent (root), bitter (leaf), astringent (stem), Saline (stem), and sweet (seed) that are lacking in one taste, "sourness". In Nigeria, there are some beliefs about the powers of garlic. In Eastern Nigeria, the smell of garlic is said to be offensive, not only to human beings, but also to evil spirits. Hence, those who wish to ward off evil spirits use it. In some parts of Yoruba land, garlic is used to neutralize harmful charms. Rubbing mashed garlic on one's hand does this. As soon as one touches the charm, it becomes neutralized. An Igbo lady recently shared her experience with me, about the fact that she has being experiencing a strange disappearance of money from her house. Whenever she kept money in her wardrobe, she would discover that half the money had disappeared mysteriously from her house, even though she lives alone. This experience had been on for some time. Then one day, as she was praying, she received an inspiration to keep a bulb of peeled garlic in her wardrobe. Because she did this, there has not been any incident of disappearance. She said she even recommended it to others, because it has worked in all the cases. These goes to show that, garlic was seen from the earliest times to be a mysterious plant.

When garlic is eaten, its odor impregnates all the body secretions: breath, sweat, urine, belches, saliva, and even the milk of breast feeding mother. The peculiar smell of garlic is due to the presence of diallyl dysulphur, an enzyme derived from alliicine, which is a by-product of alliinase. Garlic contains alliin, niacin and vitamin A1, B1,&2. As volatile substances alliin and daily disulfide easily permeate all body organs and tissues, it makes it impossible to hide the smell. The organs of the body which benefit most from garlic, are the organs of elimination such as the lungs, bronchi, liver, kidneys and the skin.

## Methods Of Applying Garlic

### Method One

Swallow four cloves of garlic three times daily, the same way you swallow tablets or capsules. This is by far the simplest and most convenient way to take garlic. It also solves the problem of the smell. However, note that anything less than the stated 12 cloves daily will give very little therapeutic effect.

### Method Two

Mash three bulbs of garlic and soak in one bottle of hot water overnight. Drink a glassful three times daily.

### Method Three

Blend 10 bulbs of garlic with two bottles of honey. Please do not add water. Drink two dessert spoons three times daily.

## Medicinal Properties Of Garlic

*Antibiotic:* Garlic is one of the most effective natural antibiotics. It is scientifically proven that garlic works powerfully against the following bacteria:

a. Escherichia Coli, which causes intestinal dysbacteriosis and urinary infections
b. Salmonella Typhi, which causes typhoid fever.
c. Shigella Dysenteriae, which causes dysentery
d. Staphylococcus & Streptococcus, which cause inflammation of the genital organs, damaged sperm cells and skin infections and blemishes. Unlike synthetic antibiotics, garlic has no side effect whatsoever.

*Hypolidemic:* Garlic is found to lower noxious cholesterol level in the blood. This makes it indispensable for many Nigerians who consume lots of fat, palm oil and butter. Over consumption of palm oil is partly responsible for case of high cholesterol level in Nigeria today, thereby increasing the risk of heart problems. Anti-Diabetic: Combined with other herbs, garlic has proven to be useful for lowering blood sugar. Those who are afraid of developing diabetes because of the fact that their parents are diabetics should make friends with garlic, as it is a very good prevention against diabetes.

*Anti-Tumour*: Garlic strengthens the blood cells that protect the body against pathogenic microorganism. If these cells are weak, the body becomes prone to viral infections such as HIV/AIDS, tuberculosis. pneumonia and cough. Garlic also destroys cancerous cells in the body.

This is the reason why people of Central Asia, who are great consumers of garlic live long. And it has being recorded that they have the lowest incidence of cancer. In Nigeria, cases of cancer, especially of the breast, are increasing daily. I would like to suggest that it is very important for our women to take garlic as much as possible. Garlic will act as a good prevention against cancer as well as help in dissolving cancerous tumors.

*Anti-Hypertensive:* Garlic has been a beckon of hope for hypertensive patients all over the world. It not only helps to regulate the blood pressure, but also helps to keep it normal and under control.

*Worms:* Garlic is also very good to fight against intestinal worms. Follow method two or three above. Garlic is also good for indigestion, as it promotes catabolism [waste excretion]. Follow any of the three recipes above. For various illnesses such as bronchial infections, diarrhea, general weakness, tiredness, lack of appetite, arthritis, convulsion and epilepsy, garlic is your best bet. Smokers and alcoholics can also benefit immensely from garlic. I have used garlic therapy to treat many people that smoke and alcoholics, and the result have been impressive. In the first place, garlic takes care of the ailments often caused by drinking and smoking, like hypertension, kidney and liver problems and also lung infections. Garlic also helps overcome the urge to smoke or drink, perhaps because of its peculiar odor. For smokers, I often recommend chewing three cloves of garlic three times daily, while drinkers blend garlic, carrot, honey and water together. The dosage is one glass three times daily.

## *GINGER: THE AROMATIC HERB*

*Zingiber offcinale* is one of about 1400 species in the *Zingiberaceae* family of herbs. In the native of Asia, ginger grows well in the tropical countries of the world. Ginger is widely cultivated in West Africa especially in Nigeria and Sierra Leone. Out of over 1400 species of aromatic herbs in the *Zingiberaceae* family, ginger is the most powerful and the most well-known. The perennial tuberous rhizome is mistakenly referred to as a root. Just as one does not call yam tuber root, so also one should not call the ginger rhizome 'root'. The rhizome is ginger. Because of differing climatic conditions, each variety of Zingiber has its own unique aroma and flavor. Ginger grown in China is often mild in flavor while ginger in Africa is hot and peppery. Jamaican ginger often has a very strong aroma. The botanical name for ginger was given by a Swedish botanist named Linnaeus. It came from the Sankrist word 'singabera', which means 'shaped like a horn'. The term officinal simply means that it is commonly available. Indeed, ginger is a common feature in the cooking pot of most cooks as well as the concoction jars of herbalists. In China, it is called shengjian, where it was used as long 5000 years ago, which was, 3000 years before Christ was born. Ginger was mentioned in Emperor Shen Hung's 'Pen Tsao Ching' [The Classic book of Herbs] which he wrote in 5000 BCE. Ginger was also mentioned in the Ayurveda, and the Hindu manual of medicine written in the fifth century BCE. The Roman physician Dioscorides, mentioned ginger in his book: 'De material medica'.

In the Koran, it is written that among the richest in heaven are passed vessels of silver and goblets of glass . . . and a cup, the mixture of which is Ginger'. In England, in the middle ages, a pound of ginger spice was held to be equal in value to a sheep and that only the rich people could afford it.

### How To Preserve Ginger

Take a walk to the nearby local market and ask for ginger, because It is always readily available in the market. The fresh ginger can last up to two months in a refrigerator. The whole ginger can last up to two years. It is not advisable to store ginger in the refrigerator. It is better to dry it and grind it into powder. Some people use powdered ginger to season their food. They simply sprinkle a teaspoon of powdered ginger on their food. This adds taste to the food as well as strengthens our system.

### Medicinal Uses Of Ginger

Ginger contains Phenols, resins and many volatile oils, such as borneol, camphere, citral, eucalyptol, linaol and zingiberol. Ginger is rich in carbohydrates, proteins, minerals and vitamins. In middle-age Europe, ginger was an important food and medicine.

Ginger's warming, aromatic properties have long been used to treat colds and flu. Ginger promotes a beneficial sweating that helps to eliminate toxins from the system and may be taken as a tea with honey and lemon at the first sign of a chill. The fresh or dried ginger also stimulates circulation and is helpful for cold hands and feet. It also aids the digestion of food. It has a calming effect on the digestive system.

It is not possible to list all the medicinal effects of ginger on the body, because ginger affects most of the body's organs. Ginger acts on the muscle-skeletal system by reducing inflammations. This is why it is useful for treating rheumatism arthritis, gouts and appendicitis. In the digestive system, ginger inhibits the growth of toxic micro-organism, while allowing the useful bacterial to grow. This is a good quality that is never present in synthetic drugs.

Ginger is very beneficial to the circulatory system, because it prevents the formation of thromboxanes, a substance that causes blood platelets to aggregate, which eventually forms blood clots that leads to hypertension, heart attack, and stroke. It is scientifically proven that ginger is as effective as aspirin in preventing the formation of blood clots in the arteries, with the added advantage of having no side effects.

1. *Fever*

   Ginger has been an ancient African remedy for fever. It stimulates the body to perspire, while lowering the body's temperature, simply soak one teaspoon of ginger powder into a glass of hot water, then drink.

2. *Jaundice/Hepatitis*

   Ginger is an excellent remedy for jaundice and hepatitis, especially when combined with bitter kola. Mix five or ten tablespoons of powdered ginger with an equal quantity of powdered bitter kola. Pour one teaspoonful into a glass of hot water and allow it to infuse for five minutes before adding two tablespoons of honey. Take a glass every day. Please do not exceed the dosage, because it may lead to over stimulation of the liver, which is dangerous in hepatitis. Some herbal scientists have even suggested that those who suffer from hepatitis should not take ginger at all. But there is no need for such extreme caution. Follow the dosage above and you will be safe.

3. *Cough/Sore throat*

   Ginger is one of the most active herbs against cough and sore throat. In this case the fresh, raw ginger is more effective. Simply tear off a finger of ginger and chew, then swallow the juice. Do this twice daily. You may not like the taste in the beginning, but you will soon get used to it. Taste is simply a matter of choice. To those who are not used to it, beer and stout or beer, taste awful. But to those who are addicted to it, it is either beer or nothing.

4. *High Blood Pressure and Stroke*

   As mentioned above, ginger is good for hypertension and stroke. This is because ginger has gingerol, which as an antiplatelet chemical that inhibits the formation of thromboxane. Add a teaspoon of dried ginger powder to a cup of hot water and allow it to infuse for ten minutes. Take a glass twice daily. You need to take this preparation for at least three months to be able to experience its full benefit.

5. *Cancer*

   For the treatment of cancer, follow the same recipes for stroke above and take a glass three times daily. Ginger has an important role to play in the fight against cancer.

6. *General Health*

   The most important quality of ginger is the fact that it is beneficial for the whole body systems. It is therefore recommended that everybody should make habit of taking ginger regularly.

## URINE AS MEDICINE

In 1996, my attention was drawn to a young eighteen year old boy, whose name was Lucky. Lucky lived in Warri with his elder brother. He suddenly became sick and was taken to a nearby hospital. His legs, hands, and face became swollen. After a series of medication was administered, Lucky got better and was discharged from the hospital. After three weeks, Lucky's hands, legs, belly and face became swollen again, so swollen that he was literally bloated. His swollen legs was as hard as rock. His penis shrank. His belly became pregnant with fluid. Lucky could no longer urinate, and could hardly walk. The doctor took a long look at Lucky and then at his laboratory report and concluded that nothing more could be done for Lucky. Lucky had cancer of the liver and kidney failure. Lucky was close to death at hand.

That was the situation when I met Lucky. He was brought back home to die peacefully. I consulted my 'orthodox' doctor friends, and they assured me that Lucky could be cured if l prays fervently for a miracle. So I did, but not exactly in the way they had imagined.

One morning, I called Lucky's mother and, in the presence of Lucky, explained to her the kind of treatment that Lucky would undergo. I told her that: As from today, Lucky will not taste any food, solid or soft. All he will drink is water and his own urine. Every day, starting from today, he will collect any urine he passes in a cup and drink it immediately. He will also collect about two liters of the same in a bowl, which you will rub on his body every morning and night. Lucky's mother did not quite understand what

137

I was up to, but I suppose in such a hopeless situation one will be ready to do whatever it takes in order for him to stay alive. So the treatment began. Every morning, as soon as he wakes, Lucky would drink two liters of lukewarm water and any urine he passed. At eight in the morning, I would come around and collect the two liters of urine stored in a bowl the previous day. I would dip my two palms in the urine and begin to rub Lucky's body with it, from head to toe. This would continue for one hour. The same thing would be repeated each evening. So it went on for four weeks, with no food, no fruits, only urine and water.

At the end of the four weeks, Lucky's body was back to its normal size. All the swelling had gone down and he was able to walk freely about, despite the fact that he had not eaten for five weeks. I examined Lucky very well and urged him to continue with the fast. So he continued for another four weeks with no food, no fruits, only water and urine. At the end of the second four weeks, Lucky looked like a ten year old boy; fresh, healthy looking and growing with beauty. I sent him back to the hospital for further medical examination, and was confirmed healthy. The Liver, Kidney, Lungs and heart were in perfect condition. I went back to my friends that were doctors and told then what had happened.

They re-examined Lucky and concluded that a miracle had indeed taken place. Very true, but not exactly in the way they had imagined. God had worked his miracles through nature. Whenever I give a seminar or workshop on herbal medicine, people always ask me this question: Is it permitted by Catholic teaching to drink one's own urine? Is urine therapy not a sin? My answer always begins with Lucky's story' And" then I would ask them a simple question: was it a sin for Lucky to drink his own urine? Was it right for me to ask Lucky to drink his own urine? As expected, the answer is always "no". Urine therapy is an ancient form of natural healing, based on the theory that the solution to every problem is contained in the problem itself, that the body contains its own healing agents.

Some people have argued that urine is a waste product that must be expelled from the system to avoid poisoning. Others maintain that urine is impure and so it is immoral to drink it. I wish Lucky were alive today to give a testimony. What a pity. Lucky left Ewu village for Lagos three years ago to look for greener pastures. He became a taxi driver and was involved in a motor accident. Lucky died. But there are many others like Lucky who are still alive and can testify to the 'miracle' of the 'water of life'

## THE STORY OF VERONICA

In 1996, a young seventeen year old girl was brought to our monastery for help. She was diagnosed with advanced cancer of the breast, and needed an emergency operation, which would cost fifty thousand naira. Vero's parents, being poor peasants, could not even afford a quarter of that amount. They began to move from place to place, appealing for funds. That was how I became aware of Vero's case. Upon further inquiries, I discovered that the cancer had gotten to a terminal stage, and an operation was not desirable. Vero's breast was full of sores/swollen and a pity to behold. I discussed Vero's issue with her doctor and he confirmed to me that Vero might not survive the operation. He said it would be better to take the risk than not doing anything at all. I told the doctor that it would be unfair and unjust to subject a patient to an operation when there is little hope of him/her to survive the operation. I told him that Vero would not go for the operation, and that I was going to take over the case. I decided to place her on the urine fast immediately. She drank all the urine she passed and drank as much water as she could. I soaked a napkin in her urine and placed it on her breast. This napkin was soaked in the urine every one hour and kept on the breast continuously. Besides this, she also did the rubbing for forty minutes every morning and night. After five days the sore on the breast was almost healed completely.

The breast, which was as hard as a stone, had become soft and succulent. Her skin looked healthy and it glowed. Despite these obvious and encouraging improvements, Vero continued the fast for another three weeks. At the end of the three weeks, I decided to break the fast. I gave her some orange juice and tomato juice to drink, followed by mashed Avocado pear and some vegetables. At the same time, she continued to drink her urine as well as the rubbing her breast. After one week of grace, Vero resumed her fasting again for another three weeks. At the end of three weeks, there was not a single physical trait of the sickness in her. The lump under her armpit had disappeared, the breast looked perfectly healthy, and there was no more pain or cough. I sent her back to her doctors for medical tests. A new X-ray of the breast was taken, and other tests carried out, all of which proved negative.

Today she is alive, full of life. She is in a post-secondary school just ten minutes' drive away from our monastery. She has been under observation all along and she has never manifested any symptom of the cancer again. You do not need to be hopelessly sick before resorting to urine therapy. Prevention, they say, is better than cure. When you wake up in the morning, drink the first urine you pass. This is usually very concentrated and quite bitter. Never mind, you will soon get used to it. Drink at least four glasses of water after your first cup of urine. Try to drink the next urine you pass after that because that is all you will need for the day. Before going to bed at night try and drink a full cup of your own urine. If you do this every day you will notice a great improvement in your health. Your blood pressure becomes more stable, your memory sharper, your libido more strengthened, your menstrual cycle more regular, menstruation less painful, and the flow more normal. Men who experience symptoms of prostate cancer or women who have breast cancer will notice a marked improvement. The body experiences a new vigor and a general feeling of wellbeing permeates the system.

It does not matter what the nature of the sickness is. Urine therapy will surely be of help, since the principle remains the same every sickness contains its own cure. When you go and get vaccinated a little of the virus is injected into your system to render the body immune to the sickness in question. Drinking your urine gives you the most natural and most potent immunization possible; for dandruff, simply apply your urine to your scalp daily. I mentioned this to a group of participants at a workshop in Lagos sometimes ago. One participant, that looked so worried, asked solemnly: 'Father, will my head not begin to smell if I rub urine on my head? I said to her, apply the urine to your head, only in the night, not during the day. Besides" if your head smells, don't blame your urine for it. Once you experience the wonders of urine therapy your doubts would disappear. For skin problems of any kind; urine is your best bet. Urine is the best skin lotion in the world. Note, however that if you wish to go into intensive treatment like Lucky, you will need an experienced person to guide you. Do not go into urine fast for more than 10 days without talking to someone that's experienced to guide you. One reliable source is the book by Armstrong, the man who popularized urine therapy: *The Water of Life: A Treatise on Urine Therapy.*

The more you study nature, the more you are struck by its mystery. While I was writing this statement, I remembered a statement made by a renowned doctor that said, "If you cure a patient from cancer, it means that the person never really had cancer. But if a cancer patient dies, it means: that he/she really had cancer." I have heard many orthodox doctors openly condemning urine therapy as useless and worthless. What arrogance! Must one condemn what one does not understand? What really do we human beings know about life? Today science has become more humble and modest in its claims, since we have discovered how complex the cosmos is. That is why the most knowledgeable among us are also the most humble, for true knowledge is conscious of its ignorance. May humility and modesty open our closed minds to discover the deeper Dimension of Life.

## THE MANY USES OF PLANTAIN

Plantain, *Musa paradaisica*, is a household plant. Both adults and children know what it is. Even though people are familiar with the plantain plant, and enjoy its fruit, they do not pay attention to its other uses. When plantain is roasted, it is called boole in Yoruba. When fried it is called dodo. The plantain plant, which is rich in lnulin, alkaloids and noradrenaline, is a beauty to behold. The leaves are ever green. The trunk is soft and contains a lot of fluid. Yorubas call it Ogede nla or Ogede agbagba, Binis call it Ogheda or Oghede, and Hausas call it Ayaba. In Igbo there are varieties of names for plantain, for example, Ogadejioke, ojioko, and abereka. The green leaf of plantain is very useful for treating diabetes. Simply boil the fresh leaves in water. Drink a glassful twice daily. However, pregnant women should not take this preparation, because it can stimulate the uterus, thus causing miscarriage. The whitish fluid that shows when plantain leaf is cut is very effective for treating wounds, especially fresh wounds. The juice stops the flow of blood very quickly. Perhaps the most medicinal part of plantain is the sap. The sap is present in every part of the plant. By piercing any part of the plant, especially the trunk, one can collect the sap.

### *How To Collect Plantain Sap*

Cut the trunk of a plantain into pieces and pound the pieces in a mortar. Then squeeze out the juice. What you have is a potent herbal juice that can be used for varieties of illnesses. Mix one bottle of the juice with half bottle of honey. Henceforth, this preparation will be referred to as Plantain solution [PS]. This knowledge is one of the hidden treasures, which many of our knowledgeable fathers and mothers keep close to their chests. The simplest things in nature are often the most important. How often do you see a banana tree and pass by without even taken a second look? Because we are so busy pursuing one material thing or the other, we forget that happiness includes opening ourselves to the hidden wisdom in nature. Human beings are busy pursuing happiness and beauty. Yet, right there in front of them is paradise. Wake up from your slumber, men and women and stop taking things for granted. Let the beauty of nature permeate you and let then let it reflect through you! The juice of plantain can be used for the following illnesses:

1. *Nervousness:* PS offers quick relief for nervousness and even hysteria. It calms the system and promotes sleep. Drink two dessertspoons of PS twice daily.

2. *Epilepsy:* PS offers great hope for those suffering from epilepsy. It effectively hinders electric discharge in the brain, thus preventing epileptic fits. The dosage is two dessertspoons of PS thrice daily.

3. *Dysentery:* Drinking two dessert spoons, of PS twice daily will bring relief to those suffering from dysentery as well as diarrhea, constipation and indigestion.

4. *Ulcer*: For intestinal ulcer, drink two tablespoons of PS twice daily. For chronic external ulcers, use cotton wool to apply PS to the wound twice daily.

5. *Skin Infection*: Apply PS to the skin in cases of burns, skin rashes and insect bites.

## *The Uses of Plantain Root*

Plantain root is very useful for a number of illnesses. Cut some plantain roots into pieces, and then pound it in a mortar. Press out the juice and throw the chaff away. Mix half a bottle of honey with one bottle of the juice. Once again what you have left is a potent herbal solution, referred to as PRJ [plantain root juice]. PRJ selective for the following complaints:

1. ***Prostatitis:***

   Prostate cancer is on the increase every day, orthodox medicine has nothing to offer except surgical operation, which is of little value. Does it means that there is no hope? Well, there is always hope. There is no hopelessness in nature. PRJ is very efficient for reducing prostrate tumor, retention of urine and other related ailments. Drink three dessert spoons of PRJ three times daily.

2. ***Kidney Problems:***

   For all forms of kidney problems. PRJ offers great hope. It promotes the 'flow" of urine and helps in metabolism,

3. ***Diabetes:***

   PRJ has proved helpful to diabetics who are lucky enough to know about it. The dosage is two dessertspoon three times daily

4. ***Gonorrhea/Syphilis:***

   If you are one of those many people who suffer from any or all of the various forms of venereal diseases, such as staphylococcus, gonorrhea or syphilis, then I have good news for you. PRJ is the hidden solution to your problem. Drinking three dessert spoonfuls of PRJ for two months will eradicate chronic gonorrhea and Staphylococcus. For Syphilis, continue the medication for four months. Venereal diseases take time to cure, so don't expect that you can eradicate them over night. And beware of herbalists who claim that they can cure gonorrhea or syphilis in a week or two. Never hurry nature. Allow the body to repair itself, because that is the natural way.

### Other Uses Of Plantain:

1. *The Leaves*: Plantain leaf is useful for skin rashes and burns as well as convulsions. Grind some plantain leaves into powder. Mix four dessertspoons of the powder with half Coca-cola bottle of palm kernel oil or vegetable, and then rub and apply to the affected parts. For convulsion, apply to the whole body.

2. *The Peel:* The peel of both ripe and unripe plantain is a cure for stomach ulcer. Dry the peels and grind to ashes. Mix one teaspoon of powder with some honey, then lick it. Do this twice daily.

3. *The Fruit:* Roasted plantain fruit is good for men with weak erection and low sperm count. Make a habit of eating one or two roasted plantain daily. If you wish, you can eat it with vegetable soup. Enjoy yourself while you improve your health the natural way. The ripe plantain fruit can be used to treat indigestion. Mash some ripe plantains to make a paste. Add three dessertspoon of honey to eight dessertspoons of the paste. Take one dessertspoon twice daily.

## HEALING WITH CARROT

Carrot, *Daucus carota,* is a well-known household vegetable. Carrot is native to Eurasia and northern Africa. It belongs to the *umbelliferae* family of plants, and grows up to 80cm high, with tiny leaves. Both the plant and the root are referred to as carrot. A biennial plant [lasts only for two seasons], carrot grows very well in its first season and stores a surplus of food in its root, which becomes big, fleshy and large and orange coloured due to the presence of carotene. In the second season the root becomes woody and less nutritious and delicious.

As early as 1500 BC, the skin friendly effect of carrot was well known. Carrot is the cosmetic herb *per excellence*. Its skin-friendly property is due to the presence of provitamin A. The root contains pectin, a glycosidic substance with absorbent and diarrheic actions. It also contains potassium, phosphorus and essential oil. Its peculiar aroma and vermifuge effect are due to the presence of essential oil. Carrot also contains vitamin B and C.

But what are vitamins? Vitamins are organic compounds needed by the body for sustenance of health, proper metabolism and growth. Vitamins are also needed for hormonal formation, building up of blood cells and for the sustenance of the nervous system. Though there are many vitamins, they all differ in physiology and chemistry. Each group of vitamins is therefore unique and different. Vitamins help to ginger important chemical reactions in the body, without which the body will lack vitality and force.

A lot of mystery still surrounds how vitamins operate and how they cause their endless chemical reactions in the body. Science has opened new frontiers in the human search for knowledge, but there are still so many mysteries surrounding human physiology and chemistry which science is yet to discover. Indeed, life is bigger than science and the human heart deeper than logic.

There are two classes of Vitamins, namely, fat-soluble vitamins and water-soluble vitamins. The fat-soluble vitamins are: A, D, E and K. These vitamins are present in fat-containing foods and can be stored in the body's fat. The water-soluble vitamins are the eight B vitamins, and vitamin C. Unlike fat-soluble vitamins that can be stored in the body and so need not be consumed every day, water-soluble vitamins cannot be stored and so have to be consumed daily or frequently.

Unlike plants which manufacture their own vitamins, human beings derive their vitamins from food, without which life cannot continue. The only exception is vitamin D which can be manufactured by the body, but even this cannot happen unless the body gets sustenance from other vitamins so as to function normally. Water-soluble vitamins are needed daily by the body and so need to be consumed as often as possible, since the body cannot store them. On the other hand, fat-soluble vitamins should be consumed moderately as they can be stored in the body's fat. Too much of them can neutralize the positive effects of other vitamins and can also cause poisoning. For this reason one should be careful about vitamin supplements. Indiscriminate use of vitamin supplements can cause a toxic reaction and poisoning in the body. It is a fact that more deaths have occurred from wrong prescription of drugs by medical doctors and from wrong medication than death from accidents, cancer, and malaria fever put together, yet nobody is complaining, due to ignorance. On no condition should you hand over the responsibility for your health to medical doctors or to anybody whatsoever. You are your own best doctor, and the best way to stay healthy is to prevent illnesses and avoid misuse of nature's raw materials. A well balanced diet usually contains all the needed vitamins and there may be no need for extra, except for pregnant women or lactating women or a person on special diets who may need supplements to booster their health.

Carrot is one of the plants with the highest concentration of provitamin A or carotene. Carotene is the most active and valuable component of carrots. It is converted into Vitamin A in the intestine.

What is vitamin A? It is a yellow primary substance derived from carotene. Carotene helps in the formation and maintenance of skin, bones, tissues, teeth, vision and reproduction. A deficiency of vitamin A manifests itself in form of night blindness [not being able to adapt to darkness], skin dryness, inability of the body to secrete mucous membrane, which causes susceptibility to bacterial infection and blindness.

Vitamin A is therefore essential for the body. It can be got in two ways; either from carotene derived from vegetables such as carrots, spinach, sweet potatoes, tomato and pepper; or from the consumption of animal parts or organisms rich in vitamin A. Vitamin A is found in milk, liver, egg yolk, butter and palm-oil. Excess vitamin A can lead to amenorrhea [premature menopause], destruction of red blood corpuscles, growth retardation [in children], skin ailments [e.g. Skin cancer], and liver infection.

Vitamin A helps vision, tones the skin and helps in the production of blood and anti-bodies. Carrot is the number one choice in any case of vitamin A deficiency. Ailments such as, weak vision [nyctalopia] especially at night, dryness of eye, inflammation of eye-lids [blepharitis], conjunctivitis and keratitis [inflammation of the cornea] are symptoms of vitamin A deficiency. Please note carefully that carrot is good for the eyes *only* when it is due to a lack of vitamin A.

### *How to apply carrot therapy*

Carrot is used both internally and externally for various health complaints. You can use carrot in three ways as explained below.

**Method 1**: Carrot juice drink: Cut 7 carrots into pieces and blend with two bottles [beer bottles] of water and one of honey. Drink half a glass [approx. 200ml.] morning and night.

**Method 2**: Grated carrot: Simple cut some carrots into shreds and add to salad or add to your meal. Alternatively, you can simply chew the carrot. This is the most convenient way as it does not require any preparation.

**Method 3**: Beauty cream: To make carrot beauty cream blend 5 carrots with a bottle of honey. Rub it on the face or body at night and leave it overnight. Wash it off in the morning. Do this every night for at least two months. You will be amazed at the transformation it will bring to your skin.

You want a youthful and healthy skin? You want your skin to take on a youthful glow and radiate beauty and health? You want a smooth, shinning and smooth skin? Then make friend with carrot. It is not an accident that carrot is so easily available everywhere in our society. It is true, and I agree, that one's state of mind matters a lot when it comes to physical appearance. Nevertheless, it is also true, as scientific evidence testifies that carrot makes the skin healthy and youthful. Do you suffer from skin dryness, wrinkles, atrophy or acne? Then make friend with carrot and you will see the difference. Carrot not only helps the skin but also strengthens the nails and hair and gives them a natural look. Such is the beauty enhancing qualities of carrot.

Carrot helps to prevent kidney stones and gall bladder stones. This it does by helping to balance mucosas, that is, the membranes that cover the interior of ducts and organ cavities. By strengthening the immune system, carrot helps to prevent sinusitis, cough and catarrh. Carrot also gives a quick relieve in cases of gastritis, ulcers and excess acidity.

Mothers should train their children to love carrot rather than coke or chocolate. As from six months onward, let your baby take carrot and watch to see the effect. It prevents diarrhea and anaemia, stimulate growth, help tooth growth and beautiful skin. Sickle cell anemia is still common in our society. But carrot is there to offer hope and solace. A sickle cell sufferer who takes carrot regularly can live a crisis-free life and grow up to ripe old-age. Carrots takes care of the complications associated with sickle-cell anaemia. Children who suffer from growth retardation and are so deficient that they can't walk, or talk or play, will benefit from carrot.

Carrot helps to expel worms or parasites due to its essential oil. For this, it is recommended that you eat fresh, raw carrot or grated. Two carrots on empty stomach for a week is effective. Note, however, that carrot is very sensitive to light. Carotene, which is the main active component of carrot, loses a lot of its potency when exposed to light for long. It is therefore recommended that you eat your grated carrot as soon as possible or better still, immediately. For diarrhea and colitis, boiled or grated carrot will be beneficial due to the presence of pectin. Boiling does not harm carotene, its major ingredient, but exposure to light does. So feel free to boil carrot with your yam or rice and enjoy yourself, naturally.

Carrot is invaluable in treating infertility. Drinking carrot juice is excellent for treating dysmenorhea [painful menstruation], amenorrhea [premature menopause], annovulation [inability to ovulate] and hormonal imbalance. nervous depression.

Research has confirmed that carrot is one of the natural vegetables with anti-cancer properties. Carotene is said to react against cancer tumours and modulate the spread as well as strengthen the immune system to battle and overpower the cancer cells. I want you, dear reader, to spread this good news to your fellow brothers and sisters. Isn't it marvelous that carrot is so easily available all around us? Isn't it great that God gave us an overabundance of carrot to strengthen our immunity? Yet, how many of us avail of these wonderful blessings. For those who suffer from cancer, I want to suggest that you blend some carrot and tomato together, as described in method 1 above. The only difference is that you add 5 tomatoes and blend all together. Take half a glass thrice daily for at least five months. Remember that cancer is not malaria, so don't expect a cure overnight. Allow nature to take its course.

Are you addicted to smoking? Are you a compulsive drinker? Carrot offers great hope where many others have failed. The detoxification property of carrot is well known. It helps in addictions like alcoholism and smoking, as it eliminates nicotine and helps to reduce effect of smoking. Carrot has depurating action by alkalizing blood and thus compensates and eliminates toxins from the system. We thank God for giving us carrot and for imparting the knowledge of its health benefits to humanity. It is our duty to share this knowledge with our fellow brothers and sisters.

## THE HEALING PROPERTIES OF AVOCADO PEAR

Avocado pear, *Persea americana* or perseagratissima, is native to Central America, but now grown in tropical and sub-tropical countries of the world. Avocado means 'testicle'. It grows well in Africa as a popular, perennial evergreen plant. Avocado has a peculiar beauty and majesty that makes any sensitive person to respect it. It belongs to the Lauriaceae family, grows from 4-8 meters height with large leaves and oval-shaped, green fruits which turn yellow or red when ripe, and an egg-shaped seed.

In ancient time in the Americas, avocado pear was used to replace meat because it contains all the nutrients in meat. When we consider the insight of the ancients in the so-called pre-scientific times, we are struck by their ingenuity and knowledge. One fact which science must be conscious of is that modern science has not made more discoveries than our forefathers. In fact, the ancients made more startling inventions and discoveries. What modern science has been doing is simply re-examining the discoveries so as to establish or disprove their scientific truth. And in many cases, science has confirmed the truth of the ancient discoveries. The ancients were great scientists in their day. But their method was different from today's scientific methods; but that in no way reduce the authenticity of their discoveries. Had our forefathers, guided by scientific, intuitive intelligence, not indicated the richness of avocado and its superiority to meat, would modern scientists have had any theory to work on with regards to Avocado pear?

Intensive research has been done on avocado pear and science has confirmed that pear is richer and better than meat. Every 100g of Avocado pear contains 160-200 calories, while 100g of beef contains 230 calories. However, while meat has cholesterol, avocado has none. Avocado protein, unlike meat, does not produce uric acid, a chemical waste that acidifies and overloads the body.

Avocado fruit contains 12-25% of fats as well as sugars, proteins, minerals, salts and vitamins. Avocado is rich in Iron and vitamin B6, and so is recommended for pregnant women, infertile women, especially those suffering from hormonal imbalances and for men suffering from low sperm counts. Those who suffer from sickle-cell anemia will also find Avocado pear helpful as it has anti-anemic properties. Avocado leaves can be used for the treatment of intestinal ulcer and I testify that it works. Simply fill a medium-sized pot with the fresh leaves, and then fill the pot with water. Bring to boil and allow it to cool. Drink a glass three times daily for one month. Alternatively, you could dry the leaves and then grind into powder. Add one teaspoonful to a cup of hot water and allow it to cool before drinking. Dosage is two cups daily.

The hypoglycemic [reduces blood cholesterol] property of Avocado pear is scientifically proven and documented. This should be good news for many Nigerian men who suffer from high cholesterol and so are prone to heart diseases. Eating one avocado pear daily for a period of three months will normalize cholesterol level in most cases. Why bother about butter when you have an avocado pear nearby? Avocado pear is an excellent replacement for butter. Spread it on your bread and relax and enjoy yourself, nature wise.

The seed of avocado pear is now a well-known remedy for hypertension. From our experiments and research here at PAX HERBAL CLINIC & RESEARCH LABORATORIES, avocado seed is among the most consistently efficacious herbal remedies for hypertension. In 80% of cases, avocado-seed therapy successfully normalized the blood pressure. I am not going to lavish precious time on arguing whether hypertension is curable or not. In fact, there is no need for such arguments. The facts should be allowed to speak for themselves. I testify to the fact that very many hypertensive patients have had their blood pressure normalized after taking herbal remedies. I am not saying that all herbal preparations for hypertension always work. In fact, majority of them do not work while some temporarily suppress the blood pressure. But that does not give us the license to make a sweeping condemnation of all herbal treatments for hypertension as inefficacious, or that there is no permanent cure for hypertension. Such an assertion only expresses the limitation of the human intellect, not the cure for hypertension. When human beings humble themselves before God and accept their limitations, then more knowledge will be given to them.

There are two methods of preparing avocado pear solution. The first method involves boiling 20 avocado seeds in 10 liters of water. Boil until the seeds become very soft. Then strain the water and sieve. Drink a glass every morning and night for two months. Those with mild hypertension should check their blood pressure everyday to avoid the other extreme, which is low blood pressure. The second involves cutting the pear seeds into pieces and allowing them to dry. Then grind into powder. One teaspoonful is added to a glass of hot water and allowed to stand for 10 minutes before drinking. Dosage is two cups daily.

In many parts of the world, medicinal plants are not so common, and they have to import most of their herbs to their country. But in Tropical Africa, most medicinal plants are easily available and they grow so close to our habitation that we even take them for granted. Consider how common avocado pear plant is. It grows all over our country, and many times we don't even give it a second look as we pass it by. Africa has many of the most potent herbs growing on her soil, and yet Africa is ravaged by epidemics, famine, hunger, starvation and HIV/AIDS. We spend so much money importing foreign herbs when we are surrounded by the best and most potent herbs, which we mistakenly call weeds. Indeed, as the prophet says: My people are destroyed for lack of knowledge.

Are you one of those people who spend so much money buying hair creams for dandruff, conditioning of your hair, or just for a healthy and natural hair? Well, you have no need to go and buy dandruff oil or hair creams from the market. Avocado oil can help you. In this write-up I will explain to you how to make avocado oil. It used to be a well-kept secret among natural medicine practitioner. But why hiding the knowledge when it will benefit suffering humanity? Nature itself is an open book of wisdom. Each person gets from it the amount of wisdom they are ready to imbibe. There is no secret in nature. You get what you want, according to your own capacity for truth and understanding. To keep information about nature's wonders from others, then, is a sign of ignorance. When you share your so-called secret with others, you will discover that it is no secret at all; that your secret is known to many others, and that you still have a long way to trek on the path of knowledge.

# CHAPTER SIX

# THE OTHER SIDE OF MEDICINE

## The Healing Potency of Sound

In the beginning was thought. Thought became desire, and life came into being, for where there is desire, there is life. Where there is no desire, there is no life. Desire became allurement, and love came into being, for where there is allurement, there is love. Where there is no allurement, there is no love. Love became word. From word came the primordial sound by which the world was created and is sustained.

The world was created through sound. The world can be understood only through sound. Sound is the master key to unraveling nature's mystery. The big bang theory of the evolutionist school of thought maintains that in the beginning, the world was a huge ball of fire. Then, suddenly, this ball of fire exploded with great ferocity. It was a tremendous bang. The ball of fire scattered in all directions. Thus the world came into being. This primordial sound still resounds at the heart of creation and is the force behind the cosmos. The big bang theory of the evolutionist schools or the creative word of the creationist schools of thought are simply reaffirming the widely held idea that the world came into being through sound.

For the traditional African, the drum is the carrier of the word, the primordial sacred sound by which the world came into being. The drum is to the traditional African as the Bible is to the Christian. The drum is the supreme symbol of God's incarnation, of God presence among us, and Logos. It is the sacrament of the divine in the human of spirit in matter, and sacred in the profane. Sound for Africans is an emotive and creative force. We can see this even in an infant responding to the lullabies of its mother, or of a snake or praying mantis swinging to the vibrational sounds of a flute, and of a monkey swaying to a tune. Through the medium of sound, the African is able to evoke and manipulate potent psychic forces.

In the Yoruba language, there is a clear distinction between mere spoken words and potent speech. The former is called *oro*, common words used in conversation. The latter is called *ofo*. The Hebrew equivalent is *dahbar*, while the Greek is logos. *Ofo* refers to words which have the power of becoming an event in life simply by being uttered. When an ofo is uttered, it goes to actualize itself. This power of making events happen through utterance is what Yorubas call *afose*. Fo means speak or utter with force. Se means to come to be, to make it to happen, *afo-se*. When you remove the fo, what you have is ase. The Hebrew equivalent of *ase* is mi-sewah, which means commandment, incantation or authority. To give someone *ase* is to give him/her authority, power, and force. In Igbo tradition, the *ofo* is a short stick, which symbolizes ritual, political and religious authority. The man who holds the *ofo* is highly respected and feared, for whatever he says while holding the *ofo* stick in his hand becomes *ase*, a potent psychic force, power and command. It is more powerful than a gun shot.

When sound is organized into rhythm, it is called music. Music is a powerful tool. No one can resist the lure of music.

Over the years, scientists and mystics alike have researched deeply into the place of music in human life. They've concluded that music is indispensable to promoting physical, emotional and spiritual health. It has being scientifically proven that music influences the circulation of blood in humans as well as animals. Music causes blood pressure to rise and fall. We now know that variations in blood circulation depend on the pitch, intensity and timbre of the sound around us. Music increases metabolism, directs muscular energy, increases or decreases respiration, controls blood pressure and influences emotions.

In some international companies, it is customary to have cool and gentle music playing throughout some work days. The managers of these companies noted that employees work with better concentration and productivity on days that music is played, while lower productivity is recorded on days when no music is played. Clinical psychologists, psychiatrists and metaphysicians know how important music is to health. I strongly believe that music is necessary to help with the treatment of mental disorders in Nigeria. It has been noted that the cases of mental illness is on the rise in Nigeria, especially among the youth. Our psychiatric hospitals are filled with young men and women suffering from mental disorder. Many of them are students or graduates. This is a peculiar kind of mental disorder because the patient suddenly becomes absent minded. He/she talks to no one but simply stares into space. The patient does not accept that he or she has a problem. Some can argue so logically about their "lack of mental" condition, that one would be tempted to agree with them. These patients are given injections and chemical drugs. However, the fact is, that this type of mental illness cannot be treated with drugs alone. This is a fact that many psychiatrists are not willing to accept. What is the cause of this type of mental illness? The origin of this illness lies in what a French philosopher calls, "existential anguish". This refers to a frustration with life because of the inability to find answers to the question of life. What if life all about? What is the meaning of the cosmos? What is the secret of life? Many of our youth are looking for answers to these fundamental questions. They look to the society for answers, but the answer provided by society is too shallow and leaves them unsatisfied. Society says; "be rich, acquire money at all costs, have pleasure and enjoy yourself, eat and drink, for you do not know what tomorrow will bring." If they are not satisfied with this answer, the youth look up to religion for answers. But alas, there is so much confusion and discrepancy in the answers provided by religion. Each religion supplies different answers, perhaps to suit its own taste. Most young people are able to absorb these complexities of life and live a "normal" life, but there are some people, especially those that have a more sensitive and subtle temperament, like poets and artists, who react by losing touch with reality. Medical examinations does not reveal anything wrong with them, neither will drugs give them much relief. They need a special and subtle kind of therapy, which is music. Our environment is so congested with toxic waste and unhealthy noise that we hardly hear pure sound.

The music played in churches is nothing more than cacophonies of organs, guitars and jazz bands, which give immediate gratification, but does not satisfy. Go off to the riverbank, to the forest, to the valley, away from the noises of televisions, radios, and jazz bands, to appreciate pure sound. Or you can sit still in a secluded place and listen to your heartbeat, your breath and your circulation. You will note that your body is governed by a certain rhythm. Music permeates your being, you are nothing but music. The body is a living entity, an intelligent being with its own laws. The wisdom of the cosmos is reflected in the body, and the body is a musical composition. The different forms of sound, the human voice, sound of nature, and the sound of music carry waves of energy which they impress on us. If these energies are negative, we become sick. If they are positive, we become harmonious. That is the reason why today, many people are sick. Medical examinations reveal that nothing is wrong with them; yet, they feel tired, weak and sick continually. Such people need a physician that can help them discover and maintain a triangular equilibrium of their energies. When sound is sustained, the vibration begins to create a corresponding pattern. This pattern is reflected in the mood and behavior of people that are present. Sound affects the pulse, breath, blood pressure, body temperature and muscle and tissue of the listener. Even if ears do not perceive the sound, the skin and bone pick up the vibration and transfer it into the system. No one can make him or herself immune to the influence of sound. This applies to humans, animals and plants. Animals such as frogs, lizards, snakes, rabbits and snails are very sensitive to sound. Even though snakes have no ears, they can perceive the vibration of sound through their skin. Modern men and women need to rediscover the value of silence. It is only in silence that real communication can take place. True enough, we are in the age of information. But what we have is a lot of information with little communication, because everyone is talking while no one listens.

It is only when we learn to be silent that we can hear the creative sound of creation restoring us to harmony, peace and contentment. Values that no money can buy.

## Medicine for death

Death is a reality from which no one can hide. Even when we try to suppress the thought, daily events remind us of it. The truth about death is this: we are humans; we will all die one day. Death shatters our illusions of power, might and greatness. A man has one million guards, has unlimited power, has uncountable wealth, and believes in the illusion that he will live forever. But death silently penetrates his fortress of protection and takes him away. And helplessly he follows. His body is dumped and buried like any other mortal remains. What a disgrace! Death is the great humiliator.

The fact that an individual can breathe and move about does not mean that he or she is alive. He or she may be dead. In fact, many of the people who walked our streets are dead. They have no self knowledge. They do not know who they are, where they are going and what their destiny is. They just live aimlessly. They are ghosts. They are not alive.

We are often told that death means the death of the body. Do not be deceived. The body does not die. The human body is composed of water, air, fire, and earth. At death, the body simply disintegrates. Water returns to water. Air returns to air. Earth returns to earth. The soul returns to its source. The body and the soul do not die. Nothing dies. There is only one life; God. All other creatures are simply sharing in the same life. Life cannot die. Life manifests itself at various degrees in different creatures. Things are alive to the degree that they are in touch with Life. The further away they are from life, the less Life they possess. The closer they are to life, the more life they possess. Other creatures do not have the freedom to run away from life. They always reflect life because they always remain what they are. Each creature flourishes in its distinctiveness. The goat remains a goat. The butterfly remains a butterfly.

The mango tree, the banana tree, the plants and the animals remain what they are. One does not strive to become like the other. Their beauty, purity and sacredness precisely remain what they are. Human beings on the other hand have greater freedom. Freedom to be and freedom not to be. Freedom to live and freedom not to live. Your vocation is to become one with life, that is, God. Your beauty, your holiness, and your happiness consist of being what you are; a person fully alive in God. When you are far away from life, then you are dead. You live in darkness. You can no longer see Life. All you see is death. When you look around you, you will see nothing but evil and ugliness, which is death.

Many people can no longer admire the beauty of nature, the sky, the sea, the flowers, and the animals. They cannot relate well with others because others are potential demons or are possessed by evil spirits. They see demons in the food they eat and the water they drink. About sixteen years ago, when I was a school boy, "As I was travelling with a priest on the Onitsha Bridge crossing the Niger, I saw the beautiful sight of the river, so calm, so blue and so vast that it enraptured me. Not able to hide my excitement, I exclaimed;

"Wao! This river is beautiful. "Heresy"! Shouted the priest, "How dare you say that! There are over two thousand demons under that water". But is that really so? There are indeed evil forces and negative powers in the world and I suspect that we have created most of the demons and evil spirit lurking around us. They are not realities, which we make into reality. Much of the Christianity of today is immature and shallow and of course shallow Christianity breeds shallow spirituality. What people refer to as spirituality today is called deity. Piety is honor, respect or adoration given to a person or a thing that you can admire and believe in. And also a person that you think has some extraordinary powers or attributes.

But piety is not spirituality. It is part of spirituality, but not the whole of it. When piety grows out of shallow spirituality it leads to idolatry. Spirituality is life; spirituality embraces every aspect of human life. Your spirituality is your whole attitudes to life, your world views, belief, and your principles. Your spirituality is how you strive to cope with the realities of life, how you strive for meaning and happiness, how you relate with others, with yourself and with God. All these make up your spirituality. Christian spirituality is a Christian way of understanding life, of relating with oneself, others and God. Pagan spirituality is a pagan way of understanding the world. Everybody then, has spirituality. Even the so called atheist, have their own spirituality.

To be a Christian is to be matured and balanced. A split personality or diseased mind cannot fulfill the Christian obligation to love, because love damages self sacrifice, maturity and balance. As long as we neglect some vital aspect of our life, and as long as our spirituality does not embrace every aspect of our life, we shall not be whole in mind and body. One important area of our life is music. Music belongs to the dimension of sound. In the beginning there was nothing, and God said "let there be light" and there was light. God uttered the world through sound. When we sing we re-echo the creative sound by which the world came into being. Music links us with our beginning, with life, and with God. Therefore, it is sacred.

There is always a need to get in touch with our beginning, our source, and our origin, so that we can maintain our balance and wholeness. This is true especially in times of crisis, when we need to hear the creative sound of creation restoring us to life. But today music has been misused. Music no longer recreates. Rather, it reflects the decay and depravity of our minds. Instead of it being medicine for the soul and body, it only excites our lower sense and leaves us empty. So often, our musicians sing just to make money, or excite the sense, not to re-echo that sound of creation that brings health and healing. Even in our churches, music does not seem to play that sublime role of linking us with life and love. Our Christian musician hardly compose hymns that reflect the creed in a deeply meaningful and transforming way. Rather, they imitate the current pop, jazz, rock and reggae music and simply weave their lyrics into them, forgetting that the message is as important as the means conveying it.

If you listen well to the music in our churches today, you can hardly distinguish between Catholic Hymns, Anglican Hymns or church of God Mission. Both the melody and wordings are the same. You can no longer differentiate a Catholic liturgy from a Methodist liturgy merely by listening to their music. If one calls this an ecumenism, a very shallow ecumenism it must be. Let music assume a creative role in our lives. Let music link us with life, and then we shall be healed, for music is medicine. The video industry in Nigeria has become a very lucrative enterprise. Nearly every week new films are released into the market. In fact, the video industry seems to have taken over preaching work from ministers, and they influence the people's mind more than homilies of priest.

Images are powerful. Images penetrate our souls and it often remains there. Images shape our mind and soul. Whatever image enters our mind becomes a part of us. The image presented on our television screens are nearly always witchcraft, evil spirit, sex and violence. The video industry has conditioned our minds to accept the presence of witches, wizards and evil spirit everywhere we go. We must not allow this to continue. Let people learn to see and experience the all pervading presence of God's Spirit. Let people see the beauty and holiness of all human persons. Let our actor and film producers condition people's minds for good, and not fear. To be enlightened is to be fully alive, and to see reality as it is. Then we shall be happy in God. Then we shall not die any more. This is eternal life. This is the medicine for death.

## VIBRATION MEDICINE

Some people have opined that vibration medicine is foreign and has nothing to do with African medicine. Such an opinion reflects a stark ignorance of what vibration medicine is. African medicine does not just involve herbs. In African medicine, the use of animal parts, music, sacred chants, potent speech, dance and touch are prominent. In many parts of Africa, animal parts such as liver, kidney, gall bladder or gizzard are burnt to ashes and used as part of herbal ingredients for various illnesses. For example, cow tail and liver burnt to ashes is said to be good remedy for diabetes. These organs are believed to be high vibratory organs, and taking them as medicine is a good way of transmitting these energy waves to the diseased organs.

African healers use words in form of chants to generate or channel energies either to relieve physical symptoms or to help maintain a balanced state of mind. These chants are regarded as sacred as distinct from normal playful songs.

There are three classes of sacred chants, namely: affirmation, remembrance and energy chants.

### *Affirmation chants*

Affirmation chants are songs in praise of God's power and majesty, and an expression of awe at the mystery of life. Some years back, I used to help out as a birth attendant in the village maternity some kilometers away from our monastery. Each time the clinic midwives, all western-trained and well qualified, had a case of labour, they would send for me. I would then join them in seeing to the safe delivery of the child. Witnessing the delivery of a child is one of the most faith-inspiring experiences in the world. I noted that during the period of labour, the midwives often encouraged the woman passing through labour to sing any song that is meaningful to her. They believed that such a song will ease the labour pains. From time to time during the labour period, the midwives would burst into songs that expressed their sense of appreciation for life. As soon as the baby is delivered, the midwives would break into louder songs, this time thanking God for the gift of life. Below is an example of such songs:

> *Who says there is no God?*
> *Let them come and see wonders.*
> *Is any wonder greater?*
> *Than life coming forth from life?*
> *Who say there is no God?*
> *Let them come and see wonders.*

In many traditions of the world, people make use of chants like this to express the impact of life on them. Dance, poetry and music are the most creative and meaningful ways in which human beings express their experiences of life. This explains why dance, music and poetry are so important in our lives. No culture, no society can live without these three realities.

### Remembrance chants

Remembrance chants are ritual chants of initiation, forgiveness, pact or self discovery. What is peculiar to remembrance chants is the unique role of memory or remembrance or calling to mind. Remembrance chants retell the story of an event or a sacred action that happened in the past. By recalling and retelling the story of this event rhythmically, one is believed to have recreated the same frequency of vibration that was present when the original event happened. An example will make this clearer. It was said that Osanyin, patron of African-Yoruba medical scientists, was on his way to the farm one bright morning when he was bitten by a poisonous snake. He knew he had to act on time lest he died of snake poisoning. He immediately began to recite the following words in Yoruba language:

*I heard roars of war in the forest*
*Cacophonies beget cacophonies*
*I heard struggling footsteps in the jungle*
*Cacophonies beget cacophonies.*
*So it was years ago*
*When Orunmila my teacher was going to the farm*
*He was bitten by a poisonous snake*
*And what did he do?*
*He quickly plucked the aporo anti-poison leaves*
*[cassia tora]*
*He plucked the ogbo leaves [hypoestesverticillaris]*
*He also plucked the alupaida leaves [uraria pica]*
*And applied them to the wounded leg*
*And within a few minutes*
*Poison became water*
*And water brought rejuvenation.*
*I hereby surround myself*
*With the same energy field*

*I surround myself*
*With the same healing waves*
*I attune myself to the same healing vibrations*
*That made poison became water*
*And made water to rejuvenate.*
*May the healing of yesterday*
*Become my healing of today.*

This represents a classic example of remembrance chants, whereby psychic forces are invoked by recalling and retelling or narrating the story of an original event that happened and by so doing expose themselves to the electromagnetic energy or frequency of the original event, and used this energy to solve a particular problem. Many religions in the world, notably the Christian religion, depend on remembrance stories of the original events of Christ's life for help and spiritual growth. In the catholic celebration of the Holy Mass, central attention is given to the retelling of the original event of the Passover, when Christ instituted the Holy Eucharist:

*When the time came for him to be glorified by you*
*His heavenly Father, He showed the depth of his love.*
*While they were at supper,*
*He took bread, said the blessing, broke the bread*
*And gave it to his disciples, saying:*
*Take this, all of you, and eat it*
*This is my body which will be given up for you.*
*In the same way, he took the cup, filled with wine.*
*He gave the cup to his disciples, saying:*
*This is the cup of my blood,*

*The blood of the new and everlasting covenant . . .*
*Do this in memory of me.*

Note that Catholics do not just recite this story. They also ritually re-enact the original actions that make up the story. In liturgical parlance it is called *anamnesis,* a Jewish term that describes the ritual 'calling to mind' of an original event. By ritually remembering the original salvific event, future generations transcend time and space and reinsert themselves into the same wavelength of the original event and experience the positive energy of the actual event.

### Energy chants

Energy chants are words that are combined to effect changes in things and people. This is done by poetic and rhythmic mixture of words and terms to produce an effect in reality. The words or terms used to produce such effects are called 'first principles'. 'First principles' are sentences that express logical 'truths' that cannot be contradicted. For example, the expression, "a thing cannot **be** and **not be** at the same time" belongs to the category of 'first principles'. This statement means that it is not possible for a thing or a person to exist and not to exist at the same time, because existence is a negation of non-existence. A statement that contradicts this sentence will therefore be logically meaningless and irrational. 'First principles' are factual statements that are verifiable and 'scientific'. While we have universal 'first principles', that is, sentences that transcend cultures and traditions and are perennially and universally true, we also have 'first principles' that are culture-based and have to be explained or interpreted because they express a particular world view. In African metaphysics, the ability to effectively combine 'first principles' to effect changes in things and people is a highly subtle and revered discipline. Hunters and soldiers and healers are known to be skilled in this art.

Below is a collection of some 'first principles' from Africa:

- *Dogs do not suffer headaches*
- *Snails do not suffer liver damages.*
- *Fishes do not suffer pneumonia.*
- *A goat that is buried under-ground does not know what happens overland.*
- *A leaf that is plucked with the right hand is 'a plucked-with-the-right-hand-leaf'.*
- *A leaf that is plucked with the left hand is 'a plucked-with-the-left-hand-leaf'.*
- *Day always follows night.*
- *One does not hear the bang of a spider's fall [because of its light weight].*
- *One cannot tie a rope on the neck of a live fish inside the ocean.*
- *Whatever goes up comes down*
- *A tree that cannot support us when we lean on it cannot kill us if it falls on us.*
- *The hand that puts food in the mouth always comes down to pick more from the bowl.*

The skilled vibration healer knows how to combine various related 'first principles' that express similar 'truths' to achieve his desired result. In the treatment of headache, for example, an African vibratory healer could positively change the condition of pain to a *no-pain* condition by combining the following 'first principles:

> *Dogs do not suffer headaches. (Who can prove otherwise?)*
> *Tortoises do not suffer headaches. (Who can contradict this?)*
> *Snails do not suffer liver damage. (They have no liver).*
> *Fishes do not suffer pneumonia.(That is their home).*
> *Therefore, I will not suffer any more headaches.*
> *I will resist any headache.*

In vibration system of healing, electromagnetic energy is channeled to bodily organs to effect a change in the diseased organ. To explain how this works, we shall consider Faraday's theory of induction. The theory states that any change in the magnetic environment of a coil will cause voltage as stated mathematically by Faraday below:

$$\oint_S E \cdot ds = -\frac{d\Phi_B}{dt}$$

This law applies both on the physical and metaphysical planes. Words, sound and music have the capacity to 'induce' change in the magnetic environment of things, especially the human body. By sacred chants, ejaculations, affirmations, meditation etc, our thoughts can generate enough vibration that affects the energy field of things and people, which will lead to the generation of measurable electrical charges or voltage. In vibration medicine, the hands are the primary instrument of transferring these electrical charges to others. As we said earlier, the energy generated in vibration medicine is more subtle, more penetrating and more powerful than that produced by, say, and a coil.

A man has a dislocation of his knee. The knee aches because there has been a change, a sudden change, an accident. The knee like is the coil. Thoughts act as magnet. Human thoughts have immense magnetic power that attracts even more than a physical magnet. By channeling thoughts, positive or negative, to focus on the dislocated knee, a change is induced in the magnetic environment, or energy field of the affected knee. The energetic channeling of positive thoughts is done by touch or placing the hands on the affected spot. This leads to a rise in voltage that can be felt as heat.

What I have been doing in this section is to re-express, re-interpret and re-present ancient African healing systems that were highly developed in Africa. Sadly, this precious knowledge was lost with the advent of Christianity. The Christian missionaries won converts by condemning and opposing all forms of African Traditional religious practices. Of course much of what they condemned was justifiable because they went against Christian principles. Such practices as human sacrifices, oppression of women, fetishism are examples of such unchristian practices. However, many other practices that are beneficial and scientifically correct were also condemned. Call it a case of throwing away the baby with the bath water. My aim in this chapter is not to condemn the Christian missionaries. History testifies to their goodwill and historic sacrifices and endurance. Many of them died of malaria in the mission fields, yet this did not discourage the others. Infact, there is no way today's African priests and missionaries can match the heroic sacrifices of those early missionaries in Africa. Of course much of their zeal was based on a narrow, culturally conditioned theology that saw the European culture as superior to other cultures, and the belief that only baptized Christians can go to heaven, while non-Christians, most especially Africans, are hell-bound unless they are converted.

This book is inviting us to ask vital questions concerning our African medical heritage. The heroes of today were once condemned as heretics. An example was Galileo whose idea was later accepted by Church and society. History is full of thinkers who were condemned for their ideas. I invite African thinkers to dare speak-up for the truth about African culture. When Christian teachers talk about the power of words in Christianity and other world religions, they are careful to use such terms as, 'sacred chant', 'mantra' or 'healing words'. But when they speak of it with reference to African religion, they call it 'incantation', a word as derogatory as 'native'. In March 2005 I attended a workshop on *Healing words* in the city of Liverpool in the United Kingdom. During the workshop, participants were taught to recognize the importance of words and how they affect us both physically and spiritually. Many demonstrations were carried out to show how words literarily affect matter. By combining words, sounds and tones in different ways, people's mood, attitudes and emotions can be altered. Participants were given different chant formulae and taught how to use them on different occasions. As I sat

177

among the over one hundred participants, I was lost in thought as I tried to make sense of the ideas being presented. Coming from a continent where the power of words is widely affirmed, I found the ideas being presented to be very elementary and familiar. And I wondered why I had to travel all the way from Africa to the UK to learn about the power of words taught by a western 'Professor' who has a PhD in Oriental and African religions. What an irony of fate!

As humans continue to explore the frontiers of knowledge, we are faced with two choices of monumental consequences. The first choice is to follow the call of love and make love the basis of all our search and pursuit. This choice promises a bright future of equality, happiness and peace to us and to our children. The energy generated by love is the greatest energy in the world. The second choice is to allow greed, selfishness and hatred to control our thinking and actions. The result of this is the reign of terror, pain and war on the world. The second choice is choice to self-destruct. May we choose the path of love, for this is the only choice left for our survival.

# SPIRITUAL RADIO-THERAPHY: AN APPROACH TO CANCER TREATMENT

## *What is radiation?*

Radiation refers to the process whereby waves and particles are transmitted through space. It could also refer to the waves and particles themselves. There are different forms of radiation, among which are mechanical and electromagnetic radiations. Mechanical radiations are waves that are transmitted only through matter, e.g. sound waves. Electromagnetic radiations are waves whose transmission is independent of matter but whose speed, quantity and direction are influenced by the presence of matter.

When electromagnetic radiation carries enough energy that can alter cell formation or bring about changes in atoms that it strikes, it is called ionizing radiation. The earth is electrically charged with high-energy subatomic particles that travel through outer space at extremely high speed. These high-energy subatomic particles continue to bombard the earth's atmosphere unceasingly. The source of these powerful rays is not certain. But their effect can be felt in the electrical conductivity of the earth's atmosphere. The sun, stars and the cosmic galaxies all emit cosmic rays which all combine to make the earth an electrically charged entity. This energy permeates the universe and everything in it. The plants, natural elements and animals, including humans, are permeated by these rays. Just as the cosmos radiates, so also do everything: the plants, mountains, hills, animals and humans. The human body is also an electrically charged entity, energized by the high-energy cosmic ray which is called the Universal energy force [UEF].

X-rays provide us with a critical look into the previously unseen world within the human body. Along with the development of X-ray equipment came the evolution of our understanding of electromagnetic radiation biophysics. X-rays allow us to extend our vision into a new frequency realm, thus extending our sensitivities beyond their normal realm.

As we explore radiation and discover its usefulness, so also does its side-effects became more noticeable. The discoverer of radium, Madame Curie, herself died of radiation poisoning. Science had to work hard to see how to reduce or minimize the effects. Therapeutic radiology studies how electromagnetic radiation affects living cells. Radiation oncology studies how to minimize the effects. The use of electricity for therapy is not new. What is new is the scientific explanation available and the knowledge of its amazing prospects. Several old medical texts listed the use of electrical fishes and eels as acceptable medical therapies. They usually apply electrical fish directly to the affected parts of a patient's body to stimulate the cells.

Vibration is another word for frequency. Different frequencies of energy reflect varying rates of vibration. We know that matter and energy are two different manifestations of the same primary energetic substance of which everything in the universe is composed, including our physical and subtle bodies. The vibratory rate of this universal energy determines the density of its expression as matter. Matter which vibrates at exceeding light velocity is known as subtle matter. Subtle matter is as real as dense matter only that its vibratory rate is simply faster.

## *What is radiotherapy?*

Modern science is a glowing tribute to the ingenuity of the human mind and the magnificence of the human intellect. Not content with being a passive observer of nature, modern men and women have exploited and manipulated nature in such a way that they are being both positively and negatively affected. On the positive side, we enjoy more convenience and material comfort. Information Communication Technology (ICT) has turned the vast world into a global village. Many deadly diseases have been eradicated. On the negative side, undue manipulation of the cosmic electromagnetic waves has exposed us to harmful rays. Our unnatural lifestyles and eating habits have weakened our immunity leading to acute immuno-deficiency diseases. Radiotherapy is one example of human attempts at manipulation of cosmic energy for the intention of promoting health. Whether they succeed in their aim is another matter.

Radiotherapy is a modern system of medical treatment whereby a portion of the body is exposed to ionizing radiation usually for the treatment of malignant tumours. It involves accurately localizing the tumour or growth and then exposing it to radiation either from naturally occurring isotopes or from artificially produced rays. The exposure of the tumour or growth to this radiation is done for a specific period of time daily. A dose of radiation is called the gray [GY] which is equivalent to 1 joule per kilogram of body tissue.

In the therapy room, the patient lies on their back or at times face downwards, depending on the location of the growth. The precise location of the tumour is marked out with a special pen. Nowadays a special computerized device called tomography CCD is used to track down the tumour. The most common technique used in radiotherapy involves channeling a beam of photons to irradiate the cancerous cells. This is called tele therapy. The source of energy used can be orthovoltage or kolovoltage or megavoltage, depending on the kind of tumour being treated.

## *What is cancer?*

The human body is composed of tiny units called cells. The way these cells grow, multiply and operate is very strictly controlled and governed by the body's inner dynamism which points to an unmoved mover behind everything. For one reason or the other, known and unknown, some of these cells get out of control and, instead of following the laid-down pattern of growth and operation, begin to grow, multiply and function uncontrollably. They then spread to other parts of the body and multiply there. These invasive, abnormal cells grow so fast that they weaken and destroy other healthy body tissues near them and then set up their own empire in the body. These stubborn and abnormal cells are called cancerous cells.

The term cancer does not refer to a single disease but to a large number of diseases. There are over 200 types of cancer classified according to the affected tissue and type of cell of origin. They are broadly divided into three types: *Sarcomas, Carcinomas* and *Lymphomas*

1. Sarcomas: This refers to cancer cells arising from connective and supportive tissues, such as bone, cartilage, nerve, blood vessels, muscle and fat.

2. Carcinomas: These are cancers arising from epithelial tissues such as the skin and the lining of the body cavities and organs, and glandular tissues, such as the breast and prostrate. Carcinomas are the most common forms of cancer. Carcinomas that resemble glandular tissue are called adenocarcinomas.

3. Lymphomas/Leukemia: These are cancers arising from blood-forming tissue characterized by the enlargement of the lymph nodes, the invasion of the spleen and bone marrow, and over-production of immature white blood cells.

## *Symptoms of cancer*

The earlier a cancer is diagnosed and treated, the better for the patient. In Nigeria most cancers are already advanced before they are detected, which makes things difficult for both doctor and patient. The following symptoms are significant warnings about cancer and should be taken seriously:

a. Change in bowel or bladder habits
b. A persistent sore throat
c. Unusual bleeding during menstruation
d. Unusual virginal discharge [especially with bad odour]
e. Lump in the breast or other parts of the body
f. Indigestion and difficulty in swallowing
g. Persistent cough
h. Unusual bleeding from any part of the body
i. Unexplained weight loss.

### Common cancers in Nigeria

The following are the most common cancers in Nigeria:

    a.  Cancer of the breast in women
    b.  Cancer of the cervix in women
    c.  Cancer of the prostate gland in men.
    d.  Cancer of the liver
    e.  Leukemia

### What causes Cancer?

The cause of cancer is disharmony. Does that sound funny? I guess it does. Maybe it will make more sense when I explain further. Cancer is a symptom of disharmony and disunity in, 1: the material order of things. 2: spiritual/mental order of things 3: the cosmic order of things

### The Material Order

The greatest danger which we face on the material order of things is our inability to face reality. Our five senses are so dense that we tend to forget that reality is bigger than what the five senses can perceive. The idea that we are composed of energy is no longer news. Science has demonstrated the electrical nature of our bodies. Electrocardiogram measures the electrical currents from the heart [ECG], electroencephalogram measures the electrical currents from the brain [EEG], super-conducting quantum interference device [SQUID] measures the electromagnetic fields around the human body. In fact, it is now possible to stimulate a muscle to contract and relax by reproducing the electrical potential it needs to carry out this task.

If we cut the body open, what we see is an intricate network of tissues, muscles, compounds and molecules. Each of the bodily organs is made of tissues, muscles, compounds and molecules. That is the much we can see with the naked eyes. In reality, all these organs that make up the body are made of atoms. What is an atom? An Atom is the smallest unit of a chemical element that can exist. Want an idea of how small an atom is? Close your eyes and imagine the tiniest particle, say, a speck of dust, you have ever seen. Now, an atom is more than a million times smaller than that smallest particle the eyes can perceive. Atom is the life-force, the stuff of which all things are made. It is so small that it was thought to be indivisible, until in 1897 a British physicist J. J. Thomson discovered the electron, a particle with much less mass than any atom. But then, electron is part of an atom. The lightest of all atoms, hydrogen, has a diameter of approximately $10^{-8}$ cm and a mass of about $1.7 \times 10^{-24}$ g. An atom is so small that a single drop of water contains more than a thousand billion atoms. Yet, as tiny as they are, they are not indivisible. Science discovers that even electrons can divide, and this can go on and on. In the same way, the universe keeps expending indefinitely.

Further research revealed that atoms normally form groups called molecules. Each molecule of water, for example, consists of a single atom of oxygen and two atoms of hydrogen joined by an electrical force called a chemical bond. Water is symbolized as HOH, or as H2O, meaning that its molecule consists of two atoms of hydrogen joined to one atom of oxygen.

An atom is composed of 99.999% light or energy. What this means is that we are made up of 99.999% of light or energy and only 0.001% of us is physical! Does that sound strange to you? It must be strange indeed, considering the fact that we focus so much attention on the 0.001 percent of us and often neglect the 99.999%. Everything in the physical universe is composed of light or energy and today we can photograph these energy fields around our body cells as well as plants and animals'. The light in atoms emits photons or information/instructions in the form of light-particles to our cells on how they should behave.

Due to heavy bombardment with electro-magnetic stresses from artificial waves: Radio-waves, micro-waves, telegraph signals, telephone rays, the organs of the body: brain, eyes, liver and kidney etc are stressed, no thanks to modern technology. Telephones radiate very powerful positive but harmful energies, more powerful than X-ray, that penetrate the brain and the organs and put pressure on them. Electric shavers, television, computers and mobile phones produce rays that are damaging to the system when exposed to them for a long time. These rays create electro-magnetic rays that are positive but very harmful to the cells, which may lead to a distortion in the transference of photons' instructions that comes in form of light-particles to the cells. The result is that a cell may derail, acting on a wrong information, and begin to 'dance out of tune' and grow out of proportion. These abnormal cells are the cause of tumours. Because current practice of medicine is still largely based on the Newtonian model of reality which sees human beings as glorified machines, it cannot answer the question: 'what is the cause of cancer?' All it can tell you is that some cells derail and grow abnormally and 'indiscriminately', and that these abnormal cells cause cancer. But it cannot satisfactorily explain why these cells derail and why they grow abnormally. But when we become aware of the fact that we are not matter but light, energy, everything changes; for knowledge is power.

### *The mental/spiritual order*

Life depends on signals exchanged among molecules. For example, when we get angry, adrenalin is released into the system, and it signals its receptor to make the heart beat faster or to contract superficial blood vessels. This is called 'molecular signal'. The minute we are afraid of something, our energies stop radiating outwards, and turn back in on themselves. When we hate other people, our work, our families etc, when we feel inferior or superior, when we create situations from which we want to escape, when we set up impossible ideals for ourselves, when we become envious or jealous of other people, we will have problems with our health. Our balance will be disturbed and we may have duodenal problems, become dizzy, break out in sweats, have allergies and be prone to heart attacks. We will have problem with sleep, and our aura becomes dim. Our aura can be compared to the immune system. Our immune system helps us to resist harmful bacteria and viruses, and keeps the body going. In the same way, a healthy aura protects against negative thought forms and psychic influences. The radiations of thoughts flow freely about as sound waves. As soon as they meet similar thought-waves vibrating on the same frequency, they stick to it and merge.

Think of an electric adaptor. It receives energy and transforms it into a controlled current. In the same way, we receive energy into our bodies from the cosmos and transform it. We are not made up of dead matter but of living cells and tissues. We are sparks of Divine energy. As we receive from the universal energy, so are we changed. We are being renewed and recreated every day. Because we daily frequent a place, we may think that we are seeing the same thing all the time. But nothing ever remains the same. Whatever we interact with becomes changed, either for better or for worse. A part of us goes into whatever we touch. It is therefore important that we be conscious of our thoughts, for thoughts are things.

One reason why so many are sick is simply because they refuse to forgive, to let go. They continue to cling to past memories, past feelings, past experiences. They derive some satisfaction from telling themselves that they are hurt and wounded. Some refuse to believe that they can be forgiven. The result is disorder and war within the body. This disorder on the material/spiritual plane manifests in the physical plane as cancers. It follows then that for any treatment to be successful, it must take into account the Spiritual origin of the illness.

### The cosmic order

When we look at the universe, we notice a certain rhythm; the rhythm of night and day, rainfall and sunshine, winter and summer, cold and heat, planting and harvesting. The earth rotates round the sun in perfect equilibrium. If our earth had been a little bit closer to the sun, it would have been too hot for habitation. If on the other hand the earth had been a little bit further away from the sun, it would have been too cold for habitation. Human beings and the plants exchange oxygen and carbon dioxide in such a balanced way that life can continue. In this system, there is no inferior or superior. We exist together, human beings, plants, animals and spirits as harmonious vibrations of the music called life.

Day and night follow each other. The seasons come and go. The same rhythm that sustains the universe also governs the human body. Though varied, yet each species is unique and beautiful. The rivers flow. The wind blows. The sky shows forth its beauty. The forests tremble. If this rhythm is disturbed, there will be chaos, disharmony and disease. Harmony is the truth of our existence. But this harmony has to be discovered, cultivated and accepted. We are blessed. But we have to open our hearts to accept these blessings. Health, wholeness and peace depend on balance and harmony between the negative and positive energies of the universe. The circulation of blood depends on the rhythmic pumping and closing of the arteries. Disrupt this rhythm and chaos ensues. Respiration depends on the rhythmic balance between inhaling and exhaling. Negatively interfere with the rhythm and disharmony erupts. What else is cancer but a disharmony in the cosmic order of things? When we are angry, resentful or harbour hatred, we disturb the harmony of the cosmos by sending out negative vibrations. If we cook food when angry, our angry thoughts affect the food we prepare and in that way pollute the sacredness of the food. Being responsible is being aware of the impact our thoughts and attitudes have on the cosmos. We are all responsible for the universe. Through the use of our energies we help to re-build and sustain the cosmos.

### Cancer: the water connection

When you see a river or a lake what do you see? Water of course. Over the last ten years, scientists have discovered amazing qualities in water. As human beings progress, they will continue to make more discoveries that make them challenge their hitherto firmly held assumptions. So long as we are open to new information and ideas, we shall continue to learn. The alternative is to be so arrogant as to close our minds to new ideas. This will in time lead to mental suffocation and spiritual stagnation.

Water is undoubtedly the single most important element of life, without which other elements would not even exist, not to talk of surviving. Right from the beginning, human beings have been fascinated with water. Water is the strongest natural force in the world, far more powerful that fire or wind. Everything on earth contains water.

One of the most exciting discoveries about water in recent years is the work of a Japanese scholar, Dr. Emoto. Emoto grew up in his native Japan where he graduated from the university. For many years Emoto conducted research on the dynamism of water. He took photographs of frozen water crystals. These photos are taken inside a freezer that is at a temperature of-5° C. He discovered that water from different environments or regions form different crystals, the purity of which reflects the state of the different environments.

Emoto's research shows that water forms different crystals when subjected to different tones or pitches of sound or music. He freezes droplets of water and then examines them under a dark field microscope that has photographic capabilities. His work clearly demonstrates the diversity of the molecular structure of water and the effect of the environment upon the structure of the water. Emoto puts some water in different glasses of water and exposes them to different pitches and tones of sound. Waters from beautiful and serene mountains were found to show well formed and attractive crystals, while water from polluted and dirty stale water formed ugly crystals. Water exposed to positive words and sounds such as love, thank you, beauty, good, resulted in beautiful crystals while negative terms such as bad, ugly, etc resulted in ugly looking and unclear crystals, while some did not even form any crystal at all.

What do all these mean? It means that water is extremely sensitive to sound, emotions and feelings. Emoto is telling us that human vibrational energy, thoughts, words, ideas and music affect the molecular structure of water. The quality of our life is directly connected to the quality of our water. The science of biophysics has shown that even when they dilute a solution to D200, which is $1:10^{200}$ they can still not only measure the electromagnetic frequency of the original substance introduced at this dilution, but they can also photograph the energy field of this substance too. Therefore, water has memory and the ability to store information in the same way as a magnetic cassette tape or videotape records information. Water keeps record of whatever happens to it.

What is staggering about Emoto's discoveries is that if thoughts, feelings, emotions and desires have such a marked, measurable effect on the molecular structure of water, it means that we too are exposed to such effect, since we are 70% water. Water has memory and keeps information. Water not only has the ability to visually reflect the environment but it also molecularly reflects the environment.

All our cells are surrounded by extra or intercellular fluid, and water is the medium through which all our cells remain in constant communication with each other on an energy level. Therefore, water holds the key to reeducating our bodily cells, giving them positive instructions and rebalancing our weakened energies.

### The treatment

There are three steps in spiritual radiotherapy.

1. **Right world view.** The first step is to establish a correct understanding of life. Life is indestructible. Each person is unique. You have your own unique story, just as I have mine. Even though we are journeying to the same destinations, we follow different parts. If we are travelling to Abuja from Lagos, you could travel by air while I travel by land. You could travel through Ibadan while I pass through Benin City. There are many routes, but at the end, we shall arrive at Abuja. The route that I follow depends on what I want, when I want to arrive and my taste. It is my decision. I am in control of my life.

   Why do some people develop cancer while others do not? Is it because they sinned against God? Is it because God does not love them as much as others? They say smokers are liable to die young, but some people have smoked for years and live to a ripe old age without developing any form of cancer, while some who took the greatest care about their diet developed cancer. Why? According to *material medica*, cancer is incurable. But what about the many who have been cured? I remember Oliver, who was diagnosed to have advanced intestinal cancer 15 years ago, and was given three months to live. Today, Oliver is over 60 and still waxing strong, while the doctor who made the diagnosis died five years ago of prostate cancer. What about Basil who suffered a mild heart attack 10 years ago and after thorough medical check-up he was given just two months to live. Today he is in his 70s and looking healthy. Louise May, an American lady, suffered from cancer and was given up by her doctors as a hopeless case. But she made up her mind not to give up, and she was eventually cured. She wrote her experiences in her best-selling book: *You can heal your life.*

Louise's story is well known to us because she wrote down her story. Oliver and Basil did not write, so we don't know what they passed through mentally, or what transformation came upon them, or how they overcame their infirmities. From Louise's story and from the stories of others, one thing is clear: these special people followed their own way. They did not get healed by following another person's way. They contributed something to our deposit of knowledge by their struggle. We know that their healing was preceded by a transformation of their worldviews. What is healing if not a transformation of worldviews?

Each of us must follow his own way. No two people are the same. You may share with me your story, your feelings, your ideas of healing. But that does not mean that I will follow exactly your way. I must find my own way. I am unique. You are unique. Though we belong together, we are different. There is and their can never be any person like me.

The greatest war that unwell people have to fight is to resist the conventional mentality or worldviews. The fact that majority holds a view does not mean it is right. Infact, Tony de mello, a well-known spiritual author, went as far as saying that once everybody agrees on a point, you can bet that they are wrong. The thought: cancer is incurable, is a conventional belief. To be healed, I must reaffirm the other belief: I can be well. I will be well. I am well. Doctors say that cancer is terminal. It is true that people die of cancer and may continue to die, but I am not 'people'. I am me. I am this unique person who cannot be duplicated. As a unique person, I cannot, and must not succumb myself to this belief, because it is only a transient belief. I must find my own way despite the conventional belief system. I must go back memory lane and discover the truth of my being.

A number of times I have heard cancer patients tearfully complain that they were told by their doctors that they must die because they have cancer. Some were told: 'Come for surgery or die. Nothing else can help you, not even prayer. Have you ever seen anybody who was cured of cancer by prayer?' It is impossible to describe the amount of damage this idea has caused to people's psyche. When a man fires a gun at another man, we arrest and prosecute him. But who will arrest a doctor who transfers his negative, evil thoughts to his patients? More deaths occur from mistakes by doctors today than from all other illnesses combined together. But who dare speak up?

The challenge before the unwell people then, is to first of all attack the cancerous cells of negative, self-defeating beliefs. It not an easy task because you are swimming against a strong tide of negative opinions. The best physician is one who helps the sick to discover the healer within. Each person is their own best healer. As physicians, people come to us and say: please cure me. We should let them know that they are their own best healers. We are only guides. When a physician says: 'You will die if I don't treat you', we are thereby encouraging that dependency syndrome that achieves nothing but fuel the ego of the physician. I remember the words of William Blake, the English poet: "I must create a system or be enslaved in another man's". Many of our physicians are practically bonded by the system in which they were trained and they can't get out of it. They see and judge and interpret everything from this narrow point of view. The great ones are those who refused to be enslaved by the system and created their own systems. It is to such courageous men and women that we owe the new discoveries in the areas of Medicine, Agriculture, technology and science. These courageous men and women resisted being enslaved by other people's systems but created their own systems. We Africans score very low in this area of originality. We will rather follow other people's systems, rather than create our own. We do not want to be laughed at, or perhaps we are not sure of ourselves.

2. ***Right focus***. Learn to focus on one thing. Think good thoughts. Don't focus on the problem, focus on the result. You can have a picture of you when still healthy. Learn to imagine what you want to achieve. What you think is what you become. Thoughts are things. See the healthy cells of your body in your mind's eye and talk to them. Talk to your body daily. Don't focus on the sickness, but on life, on health. Communicate with the good cells. Thank them for their good work, and ask the misbehaving cells to 'behave'. You are master of your body. Right focus means we think of life rather than death. This is not avoiding reality. Not at all. We know and acknowledge that we have a problem. Infact, to do right focusing, we have to admit that there is a problem. Admitting that there is a problem is different from succumbing to defeat.

Learn to say positive things and avoid grumblings. You can be happy despite your condition. Modern society is crazy about avoiding death. Society avoids talking about death, but ended up focusing so much on death. What is death anyway if not existence on another plane? The experience of death is the most natural experience in the world. At the moment of death, we shall be surprised to see how easy and natural death is, and we shall be embarrassed by our exaggerated fear and idea of death. In the treatment of cancer, or any illness, we are not fighting against death. Death is a doorway we must pass through in order to enter another world. It is not a tragedy, but a stage in our journey to eternity. There is only one reality then: LIFE. And this should be our focus.

3. **Channelling**: When we have learned to focus our attention on the positive aspect of life, we become energized. Consciousness is energy. Where consciousness goes, there energy goes. The next thing is to place your hand on the affected part of the body: breast, stomach, leg, and throat. Place your hand on the spot and talk to the cells. Thank them for their work. Congratulate your immune system for keeping guard over the body. Ask the diseased cells to be infused with healing lights and be transformed. Ask the healthy cells to keep on resisting the unhealthy cells and wipe them out. Do this every day and watch yourself being transformed. Please note that this method is not meant to replace medical treatment. You can easily do this even as you continue with your medications. It will be clear to you when you need to stop your medication. To those who have already been condemned by *material medica* as incurable, there is a greater challenge for them to discover the healer within and be renewed.

4. **Water**: We already said a lot about water above. In this treatment of cancer, water is vital. What is cancer if not a breakdown in communication among the bodily cells? The millions of molecules and atoms in nature communicate. Water is the medium through which these communications take place. For those who are too weak to place their hands on the affected part of the body for long, or those whose hand could not reach the affected parts like the spinal cord etc, water provides a good alternative. Place a glass of water in your hands and speak loving words to it. For example: 'Love brings healing', 'Harmony is the truth of my being.' 'I am beautiful'.

# CHAPTER SEVEN

# THE HEALING RADIANCE OF COLOURS

## *LET ME BE*

*Do not paint me black my brother*
*For tomorrow I may be White*
*Do not paint me green*
*For tomorrow I may be red*
*Do not paint me yellow*
*For tomorrow I may be brown*
*Do not paint me at all*
*But simply let me be*
*If you simply let me be*
*You will not need to paint me*
*For You will see me in my real colour*
*If you let me be what I am*

Colour has a real energy that affects us at a physical level. In a way colour is just our way of detecting and recognizing the energy of light from stars, and identifying what that energy is doing to the objects it is absorbed or reflected by. Our personal choice of colours reflects real differences in our energy make up, and gives important clues about the way we choose to act and react in the world. Our colour preferences show us clearly where our personal strengths and weaknesses lie. The choice of colour we make indicates our inner state.

Colour is all around us, so close that we take it for granted. We are all deeply affected by colours, more than we realize. Colours can evoke in us memories of events buried in the mind. Seeing a colour can evoke feelings of joy, pain, love, sorrow, belonging and acceptance. Colour is the window to the hidden depths of our complex soul. We all know that there are many aspects of ourselves that are hidden from us. Sometimes we are afraid to look into our soul, for we may not like what we see. Yet, we shall not be fully healed until we have the courage to face the truth about ourselves. Colour creatively links us with our inner selves. It re-binds, re-unites and re-creates. Colour is very much with us as our guide and motivator. Colour is the forgotten healer within us, the voiceless voice, and the healing ray within. Colour links us with the earth and reminds us that we are dust, and unto dust we shall return. Yes, we are fragile, mortal beings. It is when we discover and accept our limitation and fragility that we suddenly discover the amazing power within us. Our strength becomes manifest when we accept our weaknesses.

Colour refreshes, reenergizes and reactivates. It softens the hard heart, consoles the sad, soothes the weary, enlivens the depressed, calms the excited and reorients the confused. Do you often experience failure in your business? Do you have problem keeping friends? Do you have problem passing your exams? Are you jobless and need a job? Do you suffer from constant headache, perennial stress, persistent fever, recurring nightmares, irregular heartbeat, problematic blood pressure, painful menstruation or difficulty in conception? Do you know the cause of all these ailments? Well, colour knows. You know too, only that you don't know that you know. Get attuned to colour, and it will teach you many things.

From sunrise to sunset, light changes in brightness and intensity. As the morning sun rises, hues of red, gold or orange envelop the earth. Have you ever gone off to a garden or a hill and gazed at the morning sun as it rises? The animals respond creatively as the red/gold rays of the sun energize their cells and they feel a new lease of life. The Lions roar. The birds sing. The cocks crow. The leopards leap. The plants radiate aliveness and health as they bask in the rays of the sun. Each plant and animal respond in thankfulness to Life for the sheer gift of life. Human beings, on the other hand, are often too busy to notice the resplendent beauty of light. Those who live in the cities do not even have the luxury of being able to relax and gaze into the sky to notice the beauty of the rising sun, no thanks to our sky scrapers and luxurious man-made prisons we call house. Colour affects us at the different layers of our being, whether we see it or not. Every cell in the body is very sensitive to light and absorbs colour rays easily. White light is made up of electromagnetic vibrations the wavelength of which vary from 350 to 750 nanometer [1 nanometer is 1 billionth of a meter]. Each colour is a wavelength of light travelling at a different frequency or speed. Light with a wavelength of750nm appears to us as red. Red has a slow, long wavelength that energises chemical reactions. Light with a wavelength of 350nm appears to us as violet. Violet has a faster but shorter frequency that tends to pass through matter. If you manipulate red to move at a slower frequency it becomes infra-red, and if slower, micro-wave energy. Manipulate violet to move at a higher frequency and it becomes ultra-violet and X-rays. Light with a wavelength of 600nm appears to us as orange, if the wavelength is slightly shorter, it appears as yellow; if shorter, it appears as green; if shorter still, it appears as blue; then indigo and finally violet. The shorter the wavelength, the higher the frequency of vibration. Thus red, which has the longest wave length, has the slowest frequency while violet which has the shortest wavelength has the fastest frequency.

Attraction to a particular colour is attraction to a very specific sort of energy. Colour, like food, supplies needed nutrients to the body. A person's favourite colour reflects the energy that they need to maintain balance. If you are attracted to a particular colour, it is to reinforce you by supplying what you need. If you don't feel comfortable with a colour, it could be that you have too much of a particular energy which that colour supplies and so you need to balance it. For example, if you feel lonely, shy and withdrawn, indigo will only add to your feeling of isolation and will not make you comfortable. Indigo creates a feeling of aloneness, solitude, being alone, and that is not what a lonely person needs. Such a person will be more drawn towards red. On the other hand, someone who is too active, that is, hyperactive, will be drawn towards blue. Rejecting a particular colour may indicate the aspects of our lives that we are not willing to face and change. For example, a hyperactive person who is averse to indigo may be unwilling to change their lifestyle but prefers the old way.

How do colours work? Light enters the eye and directly stimulates the organs and glands deep in the brain. The frequencies of these lights create changes in the corresponding body organ that is affected. Colour has an energy we can modify and manipulate. Change the colour and the energy changes. Do you know that your behaviour changes and people's reactions change according to the colour around you? You could make an experiment with this. Wear clothes of a particular colour in a day and observe people's reactions to you. John loved to wear red. Whenever he went for interviews for a new job, he always had problem with the interviewers. They would suddenly become aggressive and impatient with John and of course he never got the job, despite his formidable "CV" John concluded that people hated him. I felt sorry for John when he told me his story. I advised him to learn to vary the colours around him. He should experiment with other colours. I advised him to put on yellow clothes whenever he went for interviews. John took a hard look at me and wondered what a strange counselor I must be, for he had never heard of colour energy. John went for another interview and he got the job! Change the colour and the energy changes. Do you often feel easily irritated, offended, impatient and aggressive? Reduce the amount of red around you and bring in more blue and green, then watch your mood, feelings and reactions change. Do you feel depressed, moody and unsociable; bring in some more red into your life. If you feel unwell or upset, orange or pink colour will help you to relax. Colour can bring life, variety, vitality and happiness into your life. As you become more familiar with colour, it will open up a world of possibilities to you and lead you to heights you never thought possible. Through colour you could express yourself creatively and be happy.

### Getting used to colours

Many of the things we do should be natural. But we have become so unnatural that we have to re-learn almost everything. We even have to learn how to breathe again. To benefit from colours, we have to re-discover our sensitivity to it. Begin by being aware of your body. Learn to relax and be still. Try to spend fifteen to twenty minutes sitting still and listening to your breathing. The first law is to learn to be silent. Learn to be still. Be conscious of the colours in your wardrobe. Perhaps you have never thought about this. Look at your wardrobe, what colour dominates there? Why? Does that particular colour or colours appeal to you? When you are happy and lively, are you drawn to wear a particular colour? When sad, are you drawn to a particular colour. Observing this is a pointer to understanding yourself and your inclination and a pointer to the solution. For example, a young lady has just been disappointed in a relationship. She was deeply hurt and wounded. She suddenly developed a voracious appetite for apples. She would spend all her money in buying apples. Her parents and friends noticed this and were very worried. They decided to take her to a psychiatric hospital where she was given some medicines to take. Yet, what the young lady needed was somebody to make her aware of the fact that her action is an indication that she needed more yellow energy to help her get over the pain, hence her need for apples. She wanted to forget and start life afresh. Yellow energy is what is needed to 'purge' the system of negative toxins and be free.

Buy Scarves of different colours: red, green, blue, yellow, indigo, pink, brown, violet. Spread them on a table. Close your eyes and move towards the table. Stretch your hand and pick any colour. Believe that that is the colour you are guided to, drawn to. At the beginning it would not be easy, but with time, you will learn to trust your intuition. Another method is to put some plastic cups or plates of different colours on a table and go to pick one. The same with ointments. You can also use electric bulbs to create the colour you want. Simply light the bulb of the colour you prefer. This creates the required energy you need. Colours are linked with the energy centers of the body. By projecting this colour, visualizing it or applying it, the energy centers are activated

## Black

Black is the absorption of all colours. Black contains all colours within itself. All colours eventually rescind into blackness. Black means dignity, mourning, mystery, elegance, self-confidence, incubation, becoming, containment, hospitality, power, awesomeness. Negatively it means evil, nightmare, rape, death, void, confusion. Black does not radiate but contain in itself the seed of radiation, infinite possibilities.

To some people, black is not attractive. It represents evil, nothingness, ugliness and mysterious ordinariness. Some see it as safe and attractive. However, black tells us much about ourselves. Being too much in love with black or too averse to it could indicate that we are resisting change. Maybe we are afraid of challenges and would not want to take any risk and so we prefer to stay where we are. Such a life cannot be happy because it will be deprived of adventure. Wearing black keeps someone safe from curious eyes. Black gives anonymity. But as soon as another colour is added, black becomes expressive, not silent. The power of black is silent.

Black can be an escape. Some people prefer the comfort of the dark night. It may indicate that we long for the safety and security of the womb. When the baby is born, they cry out because they are suddenly exposed to light. But the child would soon get used to it. Excessive attraction to black may tell us that we don't want to let go, that we prefer to remain in the past, clinging to old memories, wounds and feelings. Deep emotions and very painful experiences reside in the 'dark side' of our psyche. Many times we are afraid to face the truth about ourselves and about life. One way of escaping from reality is to fill our time with activity and work. Black could be an invitation to us to be courageous. To face the void and love the darkness. By allowing ourselves to become familiar with black, we overcome the fear of being alone and fear of emptiness of the mind. We surrender ourselves to the powerful liberating mystery which God is.

## *White*

White is a reflection of all colours. It means innocence, virginity, purity, freshness, neutrality, grace, divinity. Negatively it means blankness, harshness, blindness, shallowness, deceitfulness, cowardice, betrayal. White is the mother of all colours because they are all derived from white. A mixture of red, yellow and blue reverses to white. White is a neutral colour. White is what you make it to be. It is the colour of freedom. You are master of your life. You are responsible for what you become because you can only become what you choose to. In some cultures, white is the colour of death, sorrow and sadness. In other cultures, white is the colour of joy, happiness and holiness. White is open to many interpretations. In a way, white is red, blue, green, brown, yellow etc vibrating at different frequencies. White could be a sign of humility and sincerity. It can also indicate a holier-than-thou attitude, putting oneself above others and keeping them away. The message of white is clear and simple: you become what you choose to be.

## *Red*

Red represents preservation of the life-force. Societies such as the Red Cross use red as their symbol. Red indicates danger to life or increase of it. Most warning signs are in red. Red is the colour of activity and motion. Too much red indicates too much activity while too little red indicates low activity. Red relates to the circulation of the blood. Physical exercise such as jogging, walking and cycling open the cells to more inflow of red energy and thus increase circulation of blood. The drive to start new projects, create new foundations for business and compete with others is linked with red. Those who want to create material abundance for themselves, improve their business and increase the mental energy to survive should bring more red into their lives. Red is the colour of reproduction. In a society where infertility is on the increase, we need knowledge of the use of red energy to solve our problems. The use of red *acalypha* is recommended for the increase of red energy. Squeeze some fresh leaves of *acalypha* in water and take half a glass every night. Red clove and *Terminalia* [umbrella tree] fruit is a good source of red energy.

Red is the colour of passion, feelings, emotions and gross physical life. It is the lowest and densest radiatory energy in the cosmic spectrum of colours. It can be experienced as heat. It reliefs impotence, infertility, arthritis, menstrual disorders, and tiredness. The use of infra-red light is an artificial way of channeling red energy into the body. Infra-red is now sold in the market in the form of red light to treat arthritis. Far infrared is a portion of light from the sun. This portion of sunlight is essential for life to continue on earth. Living things absorb this light as heat energy.

Scientists have now devised means of harnessing the infrared energy to charge and strengthen human body. This is done by energising bed sheets, pillow cases, socks, seat pads of chairs, cars, office tables, etc with infrared energy.

Have you ever wondered why animals and even human beings love to sit under trees? They are subconsciously drawn to it because the leaves of trees are able to absorb infrared light from the sun and radiate it to nearby creatures. Sitting or standing under a tree is a good way of receiving these powerful rays. If you stay under a tree for some time, you would notice a re-awakening of the weakened cells of the body. You become strong and energetic. This explains why animals, such as goats, sheep, dogs, snakes, monkeys love to sleep on or under the tree. In those days in Africa, most activities took place under big trees growing in the family courtyard. Meetings could last for hours and hours on end and you would still find the participants as lively and fresh as ever. Hunters often sat under trees when tired and soon they would regain their strength and continue their journey. They were probably not aware of this radiation, but their intuition must have told them that there was something valuable there. In cases of impotence or menstrual disorders, buy red underpants and wear. You will soon notice a difference. This is not superstitious or fetish. This is a scientifically verifiable fact. Eat red food such as red beans, red pawpaw, red banana, red cashew, and other red coloured fruits. Let red energise your life.

### Yellow

Yellow is an energizing and invigorating colour. It is related to the digestive system. Our digestive system breaks down the food we eat into constituents that our bodies identify and absorb for our health and growth. The digestive system needs to keep working at optimal condition if we are to remain healthy. Yellow energy is essential for the preservation and health of our digestive system. The immune system protects the digestive system by identifying and destroying harmful cells. For the immune system to work effectively, yellow energy is needed. Yellow creates emotional and mental balance. In our stressed and restless society, a lot of yellow energy is needed to preserve mental alertness and creative thinking.

Yellow is the colour of the intellect. Students, teachers and researchers, will find yellow helpful. Yellow helps to sharpen mental alertness. It helps to sharpen the power of visualization, thinking and imagination. In schools and places of learning, yellow should be a dominant colour. You can take in yellow energy by rubbing olive oil on your body. Before you begin your studies, place a yellow napkin or towel on your head for 10-20 minutes. In the treatment of mental illness and psychic invasion, yellow is vital. Mentally disturbed persons should be made to wear yellow cloths. In cases of insomnia, hypertension and anxiety, avoid yellow. Yellow helps to relieve mental congestion, confusion and lack of direction.

For typhoid fever, liver cirrhosis, hepatitis, indigestion, ear/eye problems, stone in the gall bladder, yellow will help. Apply yellow oils. Drink orange, Lime, Lemon and grape fruits. Trees of the citrus family are the favourite tree for yellow energy. For active meditation, which involves visualization, yellow is very useful. Yellow strengthens self-confidence, promotes good self-image, and brings good luck, courage, determination and good memory. When going for interviews all business meetings, yellow is the colour you need.

Psychologically, yellow helps us to accept our place in this life. We have the capacity to become what we want to, to have our dreams fulfilled. On the other hand, there are many things beyond our control. We just have to change what we can change and accept what we can't change. We create our own happiness. We should not put the responsibility for our happiness on other people. We are responsible for our lives. Many of us priests and religious always complain of lack of time and look forward to the time when we shall be freer and have time to do what we like. But the truth is that things are not going to get better. In fact, it will get worse. We are likely to keep getting more and more responsibilities. We need yellow energy to help us accept the fact that we can take control of things and know that the challenge of our lives consists precisely in finding our balance in the midst of so much to do. We can still get whatever we want to do done, with the little time available.

### Green

Green is the colour of healing, wisdom and intuition. It is also the colour of nature, of balance and moderation. Lack of balance of the vitamins lead to lack of balance in the body. Our bodies and the cosmos are sustained by subtle arrangement and balance of vitamins and minerals. Too much of one will have a negative repercussion. The vegetables radiate green energy. Eat plenty of vegetables for energy and strength. Green is good for ulcers, (external and internal), heart problems, and all forms of infections, such as STD (Sexually Transmitted Disease), allergy, skin reactions. Rub green oil for all these. When faced with difficult situations where you must make a decision, relax and be still. Wrap a green cloth on your face and head. Green is a helpful colour for leaders, counselors, and those who make decisions. When confused, unable to sleep or agitated, squeeze bitter leaf in water and drink 2 glasses. When agitated and worried, you radiate red. The solution is more radiation of green through application of green oil to the body, and eating greens like bitter leaf and plantain. Do not make serious decisions when your aura is red. Plantain is regarded in many traditions as the tree of wisdom. In India, a person who needs inspiration is advised to hold a piece of unripe plantain in each hand, close their eyes and be silent. Plantain root and stem juice are major active ingredients of many Yoruba medicine for loss of memory. It is no wonder that plantain is regarded as the tree of knowledge.

Green is the colour for healing. We all need healing. A lot of people are sick simply because they do not know why they are here on earth, what they are destined for and what their life is all about. They become confused and find it difficult or even impossible to make decisions. They are afraid of what tomorrow will bring. Such people need a lot of green energy to help them rediscover the dynamism of life. Green gives us wisdom and inspiration to forge ahead in this life. Itis true that there is a lot of uncertainty, insecurity, unhappiness, injustice and evil in the world. Yet, we can still be happy, despite all these. In green we find the courage to face life and befriend uncertainties. Life is full of uncertainties. There are no problems but challenges. This is a better way to look at our lives. The challenges of life urge us to dare be what we are, to dare face our weaknesses so as to be healed.

## *Blue*

Projecting blue energy into the body reduces inflammation and swelling in joints and other tissues. It is interesting to note that the blessed virgin Mary is associated with blue colour. Blue colour is needed for receiving information from above and transmitting it to others.

Blue is the colour of peace, gentleness, calmness and protection. It is the colour of rest, sleep and relaxation. Have you ever noticed an office painted with dominant blue? You will notice calmness and peace. Blue does not excite, unlike red.

Blue is the colour for musicians, artists, poets and preachers. Blue radiates peace, health and tranquility. Sound, music, and water are often linked with the colour blue. Sound is linked to creation. The world came into being when God uttered the creative word. Christ often cast out devils by uttering the healing word. To the dead girl he said: *Talitha cum*. To the woman caught in adultery he said: "Has no one condemned you? Go and sin no more." Words go a long way to shape people's feelings and sense of identity. Music and poems are advanced forms of speech. Why are they so powerful? It is because they open us to a deeper level where healing can take place; a level beyond the material level of competition, greed and materialism. Blue is a mystical colour.

In times of sickness, learn to sing a meaningful song. Utter positive words while bathing, for blue is the colour of water. To chant a mantra while bathing is very useful. It brings calmness and peace. It also helps to hold a glass of water in your hand and say some words like: 'May the river of life flow through me or may the healing rays of God radiate through me'; 'Christ my light, wash me clean'. You can hold a glass of water in your hand and say: 'Talitha cum, little girl, get up' to arouse your dormant energies and power to come to the surface. Blue is the colour for fevers, insomnia, and appendicitis, allergic reactions, diabetes, cancer and other viruses like the notorious HIV virus. Apply blue oil to your body. Put dominant blue colour in your room. Change curtains and light to blue. Wear blue pajamas. In families where there is tension, disagreement, blue is desirable. Wives whose husbands get easily irritated should try to create a blue environment.

## *Orange*

Orange is derived from a combination of red and yellow. In other words, it is a combination of intellectual and reproductive energies. Orange is directly related to the large intestine and the reproductive organs. Orange helps improper metabolism without which constipation and toxicity would result. It is an active ray. It puts emphasis on health and wellbeing through proper physical, healthy lifestyle, e.g. physical exercises, balanced diet, vegetarian diet. Orange is the colour for vegetarians. In life, it is good to learn to do something physically positive. Faith without works is nothing. Orange oils, lotions and herbs are very useful for physical health. Fruit fast is capable of expelling poisons and toxins from the system. Orange colour increases oxygen, helps lungs and menstrual cramps, encourages interests and activities, releases gas, dries boils, helps in abscesses, depresses the parathyroid and stimulates the thyroid. It increases flow of milk in mothers and flow of sperm in men. It also helps in impotence and rigidity in women.

## *Violet*

There is little to say about violet, not because it is unimportant but because of its subtle qualities. As we approach the higher realms of life, words cease and creative silence takes over. Violet is a deeply spiritual colour, vibrating at a higher frequency. Violet is a blend of red and blue. In the past, this colour was associated with the ruling class, the rich and the influential as well as the clergy.

Radiation of violet is good for migraine, rheumatoid arthritis and all forms of cancer. Violet is colour of transformation, empathy and sympathy. The human heart is made to love, to care and to reach out to our fellow brothers and sisters. Human greed and selfishness could temporarily cloud our goodness. But attention to spiritual ideals opens the energy centers to the inflow of violet energy. Violet is the colour of the martyrs, the mystics, the saints noted for their works of mercy. Violet reminds us that we can fly, transcend the mundane world and join in the mystic dance of the enlightened ones.

## *Indigo*

The calming and pacifying effect of Indigo is due to its positive action on the right side of the brain. Indigo has the highest vibration in the spectrum of colours. It is a mystical colour, the colour of intuition, enlightenment and contemplation of the 'supreme being. Indigo is useful for neurotic people, which means most of us, and the use of confused minds. Because of its sedative effect, it is good for nervous disturbance. This is the level where visions become clear, where Prophecies are received.

# CHAPTER EIGHT

# HERBAL REMEDIES FOR COMMON ILLNESSES

## LOOK ME IN THE EYES

*Friend, why don't you look me in the eyes?*
*You give me food to eat*
*You offer me water to drink*
*You provide me with clothes to wear*
*But, friend, can you see the fire in my eyes?'"*
*Can you see the hunger written on my face?*
*Can you see this pining, this longing, this thirst,*
*that is boiling inside of my marrow?'*
*Can you see what my real hunger is?'*
*Can you see?*
*Friend, why don't you look me in the eyes?*

## 1. *Typhoid Fever*

### *Cause*

Typhoid fever is caused by a small bacterium called Salmonella Typhi. This bacterium thrives in dirty environments. It can be spread through contaminated food and drink. House flies can spread this bacterium. Typhoid Fever is often common after a flood, due to the easy spread of the bacterium.

## Symptoms

1. Fever
2. Headache
3. Pains
4. Body aches
5. Abdominal pains
6. Weakness
7. Loss of Appetite
8. Vomiting
9. Fever which rises each day
10. Bitterness of mouth
11. Unlike malaria fever, the pulse gets slower as the fever goes up.

## Treatment

Drink plenty of water 30 minutes before and after meals

## Formula I
## Materials:

A. 10 ripe tomatoes
B. 7 pieces of carrot
C. 8 bottles of water
D. 1 bottle of Honey.

**Recipe:**  Blend A and B together with C, then add D.

**Dosage:**  Drink 1 glassful three times daily for (NB: This preparation is excellent for appetite)

### Formula II
### Materials:

A. 20 balls of *Citrus aurantifolia.*

- Common name-Lime
- Yoruba-Osan Wewe
- Igbo-Epe nkirisi
- Esan-Ikpete
- Hausa Lemu

B. 8 bottles of water.

**Recipe:**   Slice the balls into two and bring to boil.

**Dosage:**   Drink ½ a glass three times daily for 10 days.

**Side effect**   Not recommended for ulcer patients, causes intestinal pain.

### Formula III
### Materials:

A. *Basil ocinum*

- Igbo-Nchanwu
- Yoruba-Efirin
- Esan-Alamokho

B.  10 bottles of water

*Recipe:*    Squeeze the fresh leaves in B. Then sieve.

*Dosage:*    Drink 1 glass three times daily.

## *Formula IV*
## <u>*Materials:*</u>

A.  *Eucalyptus officinalis*

**Common name**: Thunder protector, Fever tree

B.  **Water**.

*Recipe:*    Fill a medium sized pot with the fresh leaves, then
            pour in some water to fill the pot and bring to boil.
            Allow it to stand for 12 hours.

*Dosage:*    Drink 1 glassful three times daily for 7 days.

## 2. *Malaria Fever*

### *Cause*

Malaria is caused by a single-cell organism called plasmodium that thrives in the red cells of the victim. These parasites can spread from one person to another through mosquito bites. The mosquito sucks up the blood of an infected person and injects the blood into another person. As the process continues so will the sickness spread.

### *Symptoms*

- Chills and headache that come and go.
- Fever that recurs every 2 or 3 days, each lasting for 2-3 hours.
- High temperature
- Muscular pains
- Heavy perspiration
- Loss of appetite
- Weakness, pale skin

### *Prevention*

A. Avoid Mosquito bites
B. Use mosquito nets when sleeping
C. Keep the environment clean
D. Remove old cans, broken pots, etc from the surroundings.

These products act as breeding places for mosquitoes.

*Treatment*

*Formula I*
<u>Materials:</u>

    A.  4 yellow pawpaw leaves
    B.  30 leaves of Bitter-leaf plant
    C.  8 bottles of water

    ***Recipe:***    squeeze all together in C.

    ***Dosage:***    Take1 glassful three times daily for l0 days.

*Formula II*
<u>Materials:</u>

A.    *Ageratum conyzoides.*

    -   English-Goat weed.
    -   Igbo-Akwukwo nwa Osi n'aka or ahenhea
    -   Yoruba-Imi-eshu
    -   Bini-Eb-ghedore
    -   Urhobo—lkpamaku
    -   Efik—Otiti

    B.  Water.

    ***Recipe:***    squeeze the leaves in water. Make it as concentrated as possible.

*Dosage*: Take 1 glassful three times daily for 5 days. N:B: This preparation is excellent for intestinal ulcer.

## *Formula III*
### *Material:*

A. Lemon grass leaves
B. Orange peels
C. Leaves of *Morinda lucida*

- English-Brimstone
- Yoruba-Oruwo, eruwo
- Igbo-Eze-ogu, Njisi

D. Water

*Recipe:* Bring an equal amount of A, B & C to boil in a medium size pot for 40 minutes.

*Dosage:* Take1 glass three times daily for 7 days

## *Formula IV*
### *Material:*

*Alstonia boneei*

- Common name-stool wood
- Igbo-Egbu
- Yoruba-Ahun, Awun
- Esan-Ojegbuhkun

*Recipe:*    Boil and allow it to stand for 24 hours.

Dosage:    Take ½ a glass three times daily for 7 days.

## 3. *Peptic Ulcer*

*Description:* Peptic ulcer refers to a corroded area in lining of the stomach or in the duodenum.

*Causes:* Peptic ulcer occurs as a result of excessive production of pepsin and hydrochloric acid present in the digestive juices of the stomach leading to the corrosion of a part of the duodenum or stomach. When the corrosion or wound appears in the stomach, it is called peptic ulcer, but if it appears in the duodenum it is called duodenal ulcer. The excessive production of acids is caused by any of the following:

1. Stress
2. Worry
3. Shock
4. Overdose of certain Drugs
5. Eating irregularly.

### Symptoms

1. Pain in the abdomen
2. Nausea
3. Chest pain which radiates to the back of the shoulder and the waist.

4. Abdominal pain after meals5.Feeling of discomfort or pain when beans or Coca-cola are taken.

## Prevention

1. Cultivate joyful habits
2. Think positively. Look at the bright side of life
3. Pray for courage to change what can be changed and grace to accept what you can't change.
4. Avoid eating at irregular hours. This does not mean that you eat two or three times daily. Taking one meal or two a day does not cause ulcer, eating irregularly is what causes ulcer. An example is when you eat breakfast at 7am today, then 10am tomorrow, then 8:30am the next day.
5. Avoid alcohol, fried food, coffee and excessively cold drinks.

## *Treatment*

### *Formula I*
### *Material*

A. Half-ripe plantain peels
B. Half-ripe banana peels

*Recipe*:    Dry the peels and grind into powdered form. Mix one teaspoon of the powder with honey and lick.

*Dosage:*    Take 2 tablespoon twice daily.

*Formula II*
*Materials*

A.  *Persia americana*

    English-Avocado pear
    Yoruba-Pia
    Igbo-Ubebekee/Ube Oyibo
    Bini-Orumwu
    Efik-Eban Mbakara

C.  Water

*Recipe:*   Fill a medium sized pot with the tender leaves. Then pour in as much water as it can contain. Bring to boil. Allow it to stand for 24 hours.

*Dosage:*   Take ½ a glass twice daily for 2 weeks.

*Formula III*

*Recipe:*   See formula II of Malaria Fever

*Dosage:*   Take ½ a glass three times daily for 7 days.

*Formula IV*
*Materials:*

A.  *Aspilia africana*

- English-African Marigold
- Igbo-Uranjila
- Yoruba-Yun-Yun.
- Hausa-Kalan kuwa
- Urhobo—Isahrasa
-  Efik-Edemeron.

*Recipe:*    Fill a medium sized pot with the fresh leaves, then pour in as much water as the pot can contain. Bring to a boil.

*Dosage:*    1 glass three times daily for 8 days.

## Formula V
## Materials:

A.  2 unripe pawpaw fruits
B.  8 bottles of water
C.  1 bottle of honey

*Recipe:*    Cut the fruit into pieces including the peel. Soak all in the water for 5 days. Sieve and remove the pawpaw cubes. Add C to the water. Do not refrigerate

*Dosage:*    Take 1 glass twice daily for 10 days.

## Formula VI
## Materials:

A. 4 leaves of matured *Aloe vera* plant

B. 1 bottle of honey

C. 1 bottle of water.

*Recipe:*     Mix B & C together, then use to blend the aloe leaves

*Dosage:*    Take 3 dessertspoon three times daily.

## 4. *Hepatitis*

Hepatitis is a virus infection that causes inflammation of the liver. There are two types of viruses: viral and toxic. Toxic hepatitis is caused by too much alcohol, chemicals and wrong medication. The disease is transmitted through drinking water and food that is contaminated by patients, stools, sharing injection needles and through sexual contact.

## *Symptoms*

1. Fever and abdominal pain
2. General weakness
3. Vomiting or desire to vomit.
4. Jaundice (skin and white of eye turn yellow).
5. Loss of appetite
6. Discoloration of urine into orange or dark brown.
7. Whitish stool
8. Fainting.

## *Treatment*

### *Formula I*
### *Materials:*

A. 1 unripe pineapple fruit
B. 10 leaves of cashew plant
C. 1 handful of cotton seed [can easily be bought in the market]
D. All the materials for Jaundice medicine.
E. 10 bottles of water.

**Recipe:** Bring all to boil together,

**Dosage:** 1 glassful 4 times daily for l0 days.

### *Formula II*
### *Materials:*

A. 20 pieces of bitter-kola
B. 1 bottle of limejuice
C. 1 bottle of Honey

**Recipe:** Grind A into fine powder, then mix with B & C.

**Dosage:** Take 4

Dessertspoons 4 times daily for 2 months.

*Formula III*
*Materials:*

    A.  40 pieces of Bitter leaves
    B.  Water (4liters)

    *Recipe:*    Squeeze A in B together.

    *Dosage:*    1 glassful three times daily for 2 months. (make fresh preparation as needed)

## 4. *Anaemia*

### *Description*

Anaemia is not a disease. It is a condition in which the number of the healthy red blood cells falls below normal in our body. In anemia, blood is lost or destroyed faster than the body can replace it. The red blood cells carry oxygen from the lungs to the tissues throughout the body. There, the oxygen combines with food to release energy that the body needs to function properly.

### *Causes:*

    1.  Insufficient production of red blood cells. This could be due to a faulty diet, lack of iron in the food or lack of vitamins C & B.

### *Symptoms*

1. Tiredness
2. Shortness of breath
3. Palpitations
4. Insomnia
5. White fingernails
6. General body pains.

## Treatment

As in diabetes, diet is the key to treating anemia because it is vital to our body and it is very important. Eat plenty of fruits and vegetables. Avoid sugar and all sugar products, such as soft drinks and biscuits. Eat plenty of unripe plantain and fruits like pawpaw, pineapple, mango, carrot, grape, banana and apple. Take as much honey as possible.

## Formula I

(Sickle cell Anemia)

Materials:

A. *Cajanus cajans*

- English-pigeon peas
- Yoruba-Tili/Feregede
- Bini-Orela
- Esan-Olele

B. Soya beans

C. Honey.

*Recipe:*    Mix one dessertspoonful of dried powdered pigeon peas and same amount of powdered Soya beans into ½ glass of water. Add 4 dessertspoons of honey.

*Dosage:*    ½ glass twice daily

## *Formula II*

Materials:

A.  Mango bark
B.  Water
C.  Honey
D.  Leaves of *Cajanus cajans* [See formula IA above].

*Recipe:*    Fill a medium-sized pot with A, then pour in as much water as it can contain. Boil for 45 minutes. Let it stand for 24 hours, sieve and then add 2 bottles of honey.

*Dosage:*    1 glass twice daily.

## 6. *Chest and waist pains*

So many people complain of chest pains these days. Please note having a headache or chest pain is a symptom of a problem somewhere in the body. When you experience chest pains, try to find out the cause. The pain could be due to a heart problem like angina pectoris, or strain from lifting heavy objects, or from persistent cough. Besides the formula given below, any of the preparations for Arthritis is good for chest pains as well.

### Formula I

Materials:

    A. Bark of *Adansonia digitata*

        - English-Baobab Tree
        - Yoruba-Ose
        - Hausa-Kuka
        - Bini-Usi

    B. Water

    ***Recipe:*** Fill a medium sized pot with the bark. Then pour in water and bring to boil. Let it stand for 24 hours.

    ***Dosage:*** Take 1/2 a glass twice daily for 9 days.

### Formula II
### Materials

    A. Half ripe pineapple peels
    B. Half ripe pawpaw peels
    C. Ripe orange peels
    D. 8 bottles of water.

*Recipe:*   Bring an equal amount of each to boil in D. Let it stand for 12 hours

*Dosage:*   Take ½ a glass twice daily for 10 days.

## 7. *Kidney Problem*

The kidney is an organ situated on either side of the vertebral column in the upper posterior abdominal cavity

## *Functions of the Kidney*

1.   To produce urine
2.   To regulate the supply of water in the body
3.   To regulate the balance of salt in the system

It is very important to keep the kidney in good condition. Once the kidney is diseased, the whole system will also become diseased, because there will be an accumulation of waste materials which can poison the system. If the kidney is diseased, it will either produce too much urine [polyuria] or too little [Oliguria] or contain blood, or become inflamed.

## *Causes of Kidney Problems*

1.   Injury through accident
2.   Stone in the kidney
3.   Infection or inflammation.
4.   Cancer
5.   Diabetes

6. Wrong feeding

*Treatment*

*Formula I*
*Materials*

    A. Bitter leaf
    B. Water

    *Recipe:*    Squeeze some quantity of fresh bitter leaf in water. [Do not worry About the precise amount of leaves, what matters is to make it as concentrated as possible].

    *Dosage:*    1 glassful three times daily.

Formula II (See Arthritis)

## 8. *Internal Heat*

Internal heat is simply a condition or a symptom but not a disease. The sufferer experiences heat sensations all over the body or in some areas. The body is cool outside while the inside feels hot. The sufferer feels uncomfortable and unwell.

*Causes*

    1. Malaria fever at the initial stage
    2. Very high blood pressure

3. Internal ulcer
4. Insomnia
5. Excessive worry

## Treatment

The first thing to do is to treat the cause. Treat the cause and the sickness goes.

## Formula I
### Materials:

A. 1 bottle of coconut water
B. ½ bottle of honey
C. Immature coconut pulp

*Recipe:*    Blend the pulp of one immature coconut with 1 bottle of coconut water. Then add the honey.

*Dosage:*    Take1 shot every night

*Note:* This mixture is excellent for high blood pressure and dizziness, as well as migraine" headaches.

## Formula II
### Materials:

A. Coconut shells.

*Recipe:*        Burn some coconut shells and chaff into ashes. Allow it to cool and store in a bottle.

*Dosage:*      Pour 1 teaspoonful into a cup of warm water. Stir and drink twice daily.

## 9. *Glaucoma*

Glaucoma simply means high blood pressure of the eye. It is characterized by the presence of fluid on the eyeball. This injures the optic nerve and the eye lens. It is a dangerous sickness that can lead to blindness, if it is not promptly and properly treated. There are two types of glaucoma:-primary and secondary glaucoma. Primary glaucoma is often inherited. Secondary glaucoma is a complication of eye that is not inherited. An example is Iritis, an inflammation of the iris. Before treating glaucoma, it has to be diagnosed and confirmed by a competent physician who will use an instrument called Tonometer.

Be very careful about accepting herbal eye lotion from local herbalists because the eye is very delicate and should be handled with care. Never gamble with your eyes. There are good eye lotions for the eye, but only from qualified herbalists who know the nature of the illness. Just as there are incompetent orthodox doctors. [Many, in fact], so also are there incompetent herbalists. Diabetics and those who are far sighted are more prone to this ailment than non-diabetics are.

### *Symptoms*

1. Burning sensation in the eye; (tears comes out)
2. Blurring of vision, leading to constant straining of the eye
3. Rainbow color appears around lights; the person sees double'
4. Deterioration of the eyesight

## Treatment:

Consult a qualified herbal practitioner as well as an ophthalmologist.

## 10. Dysentery

Dysentery is an inflammation of the inner lining of the large intestine caused by:

A. Parasitic worms
B. Chemical irritants
C. Bacteria
D. Protozoa

It is an infectious disease common in areas of poor sanitation and hygiene. These organisms travel from stools of victims and enter the body through the mouth along with food and water.

## Prevention

1. Keep your environment clean and tidy.
2. Always wash your hands before eating.
3. Wash fruit and vegetables before eating.

## *Treatment*

Drink plenty of water.

One of the most effective remedies for dysentery is rice water. Store the water used to boil your rice and keep in a fridge. Take $\frac{1}{2}$ a glass twice daily for 3 days. Another remedy is to fill a medium sized pot with fresh guava leaves. Then fill with water and bring to boil. Take a glassful twice daily for 3 days.

## 11. *Bronchitis*

Bronchitis is an inflammation of the two branches of the bronchi that is the wind pipe that branches into the lungs. Bronchitis can be acute or chronic. Acute bronchitis is a primary viral infection caused by cold, influenza, cough, measles and catarrh. In an adult untreated bronchitis leads to acute bronchitis.

## *Symptoms:*

Acute bronchitis is accompanied by a slight fever and dry cough that causes pain in the throat and chest. In chronic bronchitis, cough is intense especially in the morning. Thick yellowish phlegm is produced.

## *Aim Of Treatment*

1. Prevent colds.
2. Prevent breathing infections
3. Clear bronchial pathways

*Treatment*

*Formula I*
<u>*Materials:*</u>

    A  Lemon grass.

    B  Neem leaves

    C  Bitter leaf

    *Recipe:*    Fill a medium sized pot with an equal amount of A, B and C, then fill with water and bring to boil.

    *Dosage:*    Take 1 glass three times daily for 4 weeks

*Formula II*
<u>*Materials:*</u>

    A.  Bitter leaf plant (50 leaves)

    B.  Pawpaw plant (8 leaves)

    C.  10 liters of water

    *Recipe:*    Squeeze A and B together in C Dosage: Take 1 glass twice daily for 2 weeks

*Formula III*
<u>*Materials:*</u>

    A.  10 bulbs of garlic

    B.  10 pieces of bitter kola

    C.  10fingers of ginger

D.  7 bulbs of onion
E.  2 bottles of grape juice
F.  4 bottles of water
G   2 bottles of honey

***Recipe:***      Mix E, F, and G together, then use to blend/grind A-D.

***Dosage:***     Take 1 shot twice daily for 2 weeks.

## 12. *Indigestion*

Indigestion means incomplete or imperfect digestion of food consumed. Indigestion takes different shapes and forms in different people. It can be acute or chronic. Though the name sounds so simple, indigestion is a very serious ailment. It is a window for all other illnesses as it leads to pollution and poisoning of the entire system. The vital organs like the kidney, liver and lungs become infected. When it is chronic, indigestion leads to Cancer, ulcer, Cardio-vascular problems, kidney damage and diabetes. It must therefore be avoided at all costs. Efforts must be made to ensure that the stomach is kept free and healthy.

## *Causes*

1.  Over-eating
2.  Excessive alcohol consumption
3.  Smoking
4.  Excessive consumption of returned processed food like biscuits, ice cream, sugar and caned products.
5.  Eating at irregular hours

6.  Anxiety, fear, depression, anger
7.  Lack of exercise

## Symptoms

A.  Persistent pain in the stomach especially after eating
B.  Feeling of fullness after a little meal
C.  General abdominal discomfort
D.  Nausea
E.  Heart-burn
F.  An experience of bitter fluid rising up from the stomach to the mouth.

## Treatment

Do not program your mind that you must eat at least three times daily. There is no such law in nature. Whenever you feel any of the symptoms of indigestion, stay off solid food for at least 24 hours. Take only fruits and water. Avoid strong purgatives or laxatives. Gentle laxatives can be of help. The leaves of *Mormodica charantia* called African Cucumber in English and Ejirin in Yoruba is mild laxative. Squeeze the leaves in water. Take a glass every night, preferably on an empty stomach.'

## Formula I

A.  Materials:

-   English
-   Water leaf

- Igbo-Nte Oka, Ofe bekee
- Yoruba-Gbure.
- Roots of water leaf

B. Water

**Recipe:**  Bring 10 handfuls of water leaf roots to boil. Allow it to stand for 12 hours.

**Dosage:**  1 glassful thrice for2 weeks

## Formula II
### Materials:

A. 10 bulbs of garlic
B. 2 bottles of Coconut water
C. 8 bottles of water

**Recipe:**  Peel the garlic and soak in C for 5 days. Then add B and boil for 15 minutes.

**Dosage:**  Take 1 shot twice daily for 4 weeks.

## Formula III
### Materials:

A. Leaves of *Vernonia amygdalina*

- English
- Bitter leaf

- Igbo—Onugbu
- Yoruba-Ewuro

**Recipe:**     Simply squeeze some quantity of bitter leaf in water.

**Dosage:**     Take 1 glassful three times daily

*Note:* This preparation is good for insomnia.

## 13. *Ulcer [External]*

External ulcer refers to a wound that refuses to heal in spite of all treatments. This may be due to a deficiency in the system or a chronic infection or disease, such as Diabetes.

## *Treatment*

## *Formula I*

Cut and dry some stems of bitter leaf, mango and cashew plants and burn into charcoal. Grind the charcoal into powder, sprinkle on the wound and cover with cotton wool. Do this twice a day. After one week of application, you will see that your wound is nearly healed. Continue the same application until the wound heals completely.

## *Formula II*

Refer to the many uses of pawpaw

## 14. *Scabies*

Scabies is a contagious infection of the skin caused by the itch mite. The mite thrives in such places as the hair, fingers, wrists, armpit, thighs and soles of the feet. From there it spreads to the whole body, causing a terrible itch.

### *Treatment*

### **Materials:**

    A. ½ bottle of kerosene
    B. ½ bottle of vegetable oil

   *Recipe:*   Mix the two together and stir very well, How to use: Apply to the affected area three times a day. The itch often disappears within 2 hours. You may not like the smell of kerosene but it is more endurable than the itch.

## 15. *Lumbago*

Lumbago means low back pain. This pain is felt on the lower back. It can be so painful, that one finds it so difficult to walk, stand or sit for some time.

### *Causes*

    A. Incorrect sitting or lying position
    B. Lifting very heavy objects

C. Injuries to the spine through accident

D. Arthritis

**Treatment:** See 'Arthritis'

## 16. *Stroke*

Stroke is technically called apoplexy. Stroke means the stoppage of blood supply to a part of the brain, leading to complete or partial paralysis.

## *Causes*

A. Untreated or undiagnosed hypertension

B. A blood clot in a part of the brain, blocking blood supply to the artery

C. Clotting of the arteries

D. Bursting open of a blood vessel in the brain

## *Symptoms*

1. Breathing becomes difficult e.g. in asthma.

2. Skin becomes wet and sticky to the touch

3. Speech becomes difficult and inaudible

4. Paralysis of part of the body from head to foot or of the whole body.

5. Unconsciousness

## *Prevention*

The best way to prevent strokes is to control your blood pressure. Anyone who is forty years and above should consider him/herself a potential hypertension patient and take all necessary precautions. Check your blood pressure at least once a week. Take as little salt as possible. Cultivate a positive attitude to life. Forgive those who offended you. Do regular physical exercises. Be honest with yourself, your fellow human beings and with God. Drink plenty of water especially early in the morning and before going to bed at night.

### Treatment

For the uses of bitter leaf plant for stroke. See the "Health benefits of bitter leaf."

### Formula I

### Materials:

    A.  Fresh pawpaw leaves
    B.  Fresh leaves of Avocado pear
    C.  Water

    **Recipe:**    Put an equal amount of A & B in a medium sized pot. Then fill the pot with water. Bring to boil.

    **Dosage:**    Take1 glass three times a day for 2 months.

*How to make a stroke lotion*

This preparation is for external use only.

## *Materials:*

   A.  Dried pawpaw leaves

   B.  Palm-kernel oil

   ***Recipe:***    A Mix 6 tablespoonful of the dried powdered pawpaw leaves with 1/2 a glass of palm-kernel oil and apply to the affected parts twice a day

## 17. *Measles*

An acute infectious disease caused by a virus. It often affects infants and adolescents. The good news about measles is that it strikes only once, after which the body becomes immune to it for life.

### *Symptoms*

-  Cough, catarrh and sore throat
-  Very high fever (as high as 104°f).
-  Eyes turn red, runny-nose
-  Bloody rashes appear on face and nose, and spread to other parts of the body.

### *Treatment*

## *Material:*

A. *Cajanus cajans*

- English—Pigeon peas
- Igbo-Fiofio
- Yoruba-Feregede
- Esan-Olele

***Recipe:***     Fill a medium sized pot with the fresh leaves, then fill pot with water and bring to boil.

***How to use:*** Use two liters out of the preparation to bathe every night for 5 days. Drink ½ a glass of the preparation twice a day for 5 days.

## 18. *Insomnia*

Insomnia means difficulty in sleeping or inability to sleep for a long duration. Those who suffer from insomnia can hardly sleep for four hours at a time.

## *Causes*

1. ***Over-Eating And Hunger***
   These are two extremes to be avoided. Overeating, especially at night can make sleeping difficult because the system needs extra time to digest the food. On the other hand, hunger causes lack of concentration and discomfort, making sleep difficult.

2. *Pain and Fever*

   Pain in any part of the body can prevent sleep. After all, no one sleeps when his house is on fire. Those who suffer from toothache will better understand what I mean.

3. *Worry, Anxiety and Fear*

   Uncertainty brings insecurity; insecurity brings worry; worry brings anxiety; anxiety brings fear. The chain is endless. Sleep requires peace of mind and calmness. Therefore absence of these causes insomnia.

## *Prevention*

1. *Comfortable Bed*

   A good bed is one with solid foam and strong springs or flat wood. The modern day cabinet beds are better than spring beds. Make your bedroom clean, cool and fresh. How can you sleep well if your bedroom is stuffy, smoky or dirty or is full of cockroaches and mosquitoes? Some people can wear very expensive clothes and ornaments, but do not have a comfortable bed. What a shame! We must learn to get our priorities right.

2. *Physical Exercise*

   Physical exercise is essential to health. Exercise promotes sweating and proper circulation of blood in the system. Those who do office work that requires sitting in one place for long hours often experience insomnia. Be sure to do some exercise that will make you sweat. Skipping or jump roping is a good form of exercise for busy people. All you need is a jumping rope. You can jump up to 50 to 100 times to begin with. Do not go to bed immediately after dinner.

3. **Relaxation**

We modern Africans are often tempted to keep working until the body finally breaks down. Many of us do not understand or listen to our body. As long as there is no pain, or as long as the pain is endurable, we go on managing until we finally break down. It is high time we recognize the importance of rest and allow our body to renew itself.

4. **Prompt Rising**

Be prompt when you wake up in the morning. Never take sleeping drugs because they have a negative effect on you. Think of others and try to do something to make others happy. Share some of your problems with friends that have the same things in common as you do.

## Treatment

## Formula I

A simple remedy for Insomnia is Onion. Simply chew a small bulb of Onion before you go to bed every night. [If you or your partner does not like the smell, try formula II below]

## Formula II

Squeeze some fresh bitter leaf in water and take 2 glassfuls every night.

## 19. *Jaundice*

Jaundice is a condition not a disease. It is a condition characterized by a rise in blood bilirubin level. This is referred to as hyperbilirubin anemia.

### *Types Of Jaundice:*

**A. Obstructive jaundice**
An obstruction in the biliary track or bile ducts that makes it difficult or impossible for the liver to excrete bilirubin.

**B. Haemolytic Jaundice**
An excessive disintegration of red blood cells with the liberation of contained hemoglobin.

**C. Hepatocellular Jaundice**
This is a toxic or ineffective damage of the liver cells.

**D. Acholuric Jaundice**

This Jaundice does not have bile in the urine.

### *Symptoms*

1. Yellowish skin, especially the eyes, palms and tissues as a result of raised bilirubin level
2. Dark brown or yellowish urine.
3. Whitish stools due to inability of the liver to excrete bilirubin.
4. Itching all over the body which can be very severe.

## Treatment

### Materials:

A. 50 pieces of Bitter kola
B. Honey

**Recipe:** Cut into tiny pieces and allow to dry, then grind into powder.

**How to use:** Mix one tea spoonful of the powder with some honey to make a paste, then lick.

**Duration:** Three times daily for 6 weeks.

## Formula II
### Materials:

A. 20 lemon leaves
B. 20 lime leaves
C. 4 yellow pawpaw leaves
D. 4 pods of Capsicum frutescens

English-Birds pepper,
African red pepper
Igbo-Ose, Ose oyibo
Yoruba-Ata eiye,
Hausa-Balkono
Benin-Isie

*Recipe:*      Bring to boil in 10 bottles of water.

*Dosage*:      Take 1 glassful 4 times daily for 5 days.

## 20. *Migraine*

Migraine is a persistent headache that is often localized on one side of the head. It is most common among adolescents between ages of 10 and 20. Migraine tends to be more common in women than in men.

Symptoms

1. Loss of sensation in the limbs
2. Persistent headache for hours or days
3. Vomiting and nausea
4. Nasal irritation and peculiar smell

### *Prevention*

1. Listen to your body. Avoid foods that your body does not want. Note if your headache follows the consumption of a certain kind of food. If so, avoid such foods.
2. Avoid alcoholic drinks, especially at night.
3. Avoid taking heavy meal at night. If you cannot have your upper/dinner before 7:30 p.m., forget it.

### *Treatment*

Endeavour to drink 3 to 4 cups of water on an empty stomach in morning, and before going to bed at night. Avoid drinking water in between meals or at least as little as possible.

### Formula I
### Materials

1. *Newbouldia laevis*

   English-Fertility plant
   Igbo-Ogirishi
   Yoruba-Akoko
   Esan-Uhkimi

**Recipe:** Fill a medium sized pot with the fresh bark, add water and bring to boil. Allow it to stand for 12 hours.

**How to use:** Use the preparation to wash your face and head every morning and night. Drink ½ a glass twice daily for 6 days.

### Formula II

### Materials:

A. 5 bulbs of garlic
B. 5 bulbs of onions
C. 2 bottles of water

*Recipe:*    Boil A and B in C

*How to use:* Use to wash your face and head and drink 1/2 a glass on an empty stomach every morning.

## 21. *Epilepsy*

Epilepsy is a condition caused by an abnormal electrical discharge in the brain, leading to severe or mild fits and partial or complete loss of consciousness.

### *Causes*

1. Disordered or abnormal electrical discharge by brain cells
2. Severe injury to the brain during an accident
3. Damage to the nervous system in an accident
4. Infantile injury, for example, a child falling from a high bed thus injuring the spine or brain, the result of which may not manifest until the child is grown up.
5. Chronic constipation, indigestion and food poisoning can lead to epilepsy in a child
6. Infection during childhood

### *Precautions*

1. If you or your child manifests a symptom of fits of any kind, report promptly to a specialist. Do not presume that the problem will go away on its own.
2. Proper rest is needed. Eat nourishing food, such as fruits and vegetables. Avoid constipation or indigestion. Drink

plenty of water, especially in the morning, three to four hours before breakfast.

3. If you must drive, be sure that you never drive alone.
4. Never go swimming. This could be very dangerous.
5. Epileptic fits are detrimental to pregnancy. Extra care should be taken during pregnancy.
6. Avoid processed and refined food such as sugar, biscuits, cheese, ice cream, and soft drinks.
7. Avoid alcoholic drinks

### Types of Epilepsy

Epilepsy can be divided into two types: minor and major.

### Minor Epilepsy

**Description:** There is a brief blurring of consciousness. The person becomes absent minded, and begins to stare into space. The lips, eyelids and head twist slightly. The person may smack the lips, move the mouth as if they are chewing something, and make odd noises. They may stand in fixed position or may gently sit on the ground. In some cases the person walks off absent mindedly, similar to sleep walking.

### What to do

1. Do not be scared or panicky. Be kind, charitable and helpful to that person who needs your care.
2. Help him/her to sit quietly in a place and be still.

3. Stay with the victim. Do not begin to ask questions. Never pour water on him/her.

4. Let the victim rest for the rest of the day.

### Major Epilepsy

A recurrent major disturbance of brain activity leading to violent seizures and loss of consciousness. Attack begins by the patient's letting out a nervous cry and suddenly falling unconscious. The patient becomes rigid and arches the back. Breathing may cease. The lips turn blue and the face and neck become congested. This is followed by vigorous fits, with jaws clenched and a noisy breathing. Foamy saliva drops from the mouth. The patient bites the lips, making them to bleed. After some time the person calms down, the muscles relaxes, breathing becomes normal and he or she regains consciousness. On regaining consciousness, the patient may manifest strange and abnormal behavior, before falling into a deep sleep.

### Treatments

### Formula I
### Materials:

A. *Alstonia boneei*

English—Stool wood
Igbo-Egbu
Yoruba: Ahun
Esan-Ojegbukhun

B. *Jartropha curcas*

English-Pig nut
Igbo-Olulu-idu
Hausa—Dazugu
Yoruba-Botuje, Lapalapa

C. *Newbouldia laevis*

English-Fertility plant
Igbo-Ogirishi
Yoruba-Akoko
Esan-llkhimi

**Recipe:**   Fill a medium sized pot with an equal amount of the roots of A, B, and C and bring to boil. Allow it to stand for 1 hour before drinking.

**Dosage:**   Take ½ a glass three times daily for 2 months.

## Formula II

A. *Jartropha curcas* [Pig nut]
B. 20 Tobacco leaves
C. 8 bulbs of garlic
D. 10liters of water

**Recipe**:   Cut the root of A into pieces. Measure 20 handful of the pieces and bring them to boil together with B and C. Allow it to stand for 12 hours.

**Dosage:**   Take ½ a glass twice daily.

## 22. *Piles*

Also called hemorrhoids, piles occur when varicose veins form around the anus. When these veins are formed outside the anal sphincter, they are called external hemorrhoids. When they are formed inside the anal sphincter, they are called internal hemorrhoids.

### *Treatment*

A.  Avoid refined and sugary foods such as, biscuits, ice cream and soft drinks. Drink up to four cups of water on an empty stomach every morning.

### *Formula I*
### *Materials:*

2 Irish potatoes

**Recipe:**   Boil the 2 potatoes for 10 minutes

**How to use:** Eat the 2 half-boiled potatoes, peels inclusive. Do this every night for 5 days

### *Formula II*
### *Materials*

A.  Neem tree or Dogoyaro Plant
B.  8 bottles of water

*Recipe:* Squeeze some quantity of the leaves in B. Dosage: Take 1 glassful twice daily.

## 23. *Depression*

Depression is a form of mental disorder characterized by periods of prolonged sadness, gloom and negative feelings. The patient feels insecure, helpless, uncertain, lonely and discouraged. We all feel depressed from time to time. That is natural enough. However, when it occurs regularly and frequently and lasts for prolonged periods, it becomes a disorder. The victim finds it difficult to sleep and experiences loss of appetite. Hobbies like reading, writing or walking becomes uninteresting. The person feels intensely lonely, yet does not wish to be with others. Thoughts of illness, suicide and death preoccupy the mind.

## *Causes*

1. *Emotional Stress*

   In these days of harsh economic realities, insecurity and violence, emotional stress is a common experience. Some people are over ambitious, pursuing many things at a time. Eagerness to succeed in life, failure to achieve the aim one sets for oneself, hatred in the family, insecurity, and fear can cause emotional stress leading to depression in some people.

2. *Drug Abuse*

   Persistent use of certain drugs like fertility drugs, sedatives, and slimming drugs can lead to depression. Alcoholism can also lead to depression.

3. *Heredity*

   Some ancient Greek scientists linked depression with liver problems. They argued that depression occurs when bilirubin cannot escape from the liver or when there is insufficient bile. Some people by birth are genetically prone to depression.

4. *Environment*

   Human beings are products of their environment. Our climate and vegetation contribute in some measure to our happiness and sense of well-being. Those who live in a certain kind of environment, for example, excessively and persistently cold weather, are more prone to depression than those who live in warm climates.

5. *Society*

   In societies where communal values such as a sense of brotherliness, tolerance, mindfulness, care and concern for the person flourish, cases of depression are rare.

## *Treatment*

1. *Love And Care*

   Depressed people need love and care. They need understanding and encouragement. Our Christian faith demands that we show this kind of love to our depressed brothers and sisters, "for I was hungry and you gave me something to eat, I was thirsty and you gave me something to drink, I was a stranger and you invited me in"[Mt 25:35]

2. *Understanding*

   Depressed people need persons who will understand, encourage and understand their condition, so depression will not pass judgment on them. A simple word of consolation is better than long sermons. Avoid preaching to a depressed person.

### 3. Seek help

Seek the company of those who will help you. Never give in to your mood. Remember that you cannot make an objective decision when you are in such a mood. Trust in God's help.

## Herbal Remedies

### Formula I
### Material

Basil *ocinum*
English scent leaves
Igbo-Nchanwu
Yoruba-Efirin

**Recipe:** Fill a medium sized pot with the fresh leaves and pour in some water. Bring to boil.

**Dosage:** Take ½ a glass 4 times daily. This preparation should always be taken hot.

### Formula II
### Materials

1. peels of lime (10 handfuls)
2. peels of lemon (10 handfuls)

3. peels of grape (10 handfuls)
4. 5 bulbs of garlic
5. 10liters of water

*Recipe:*    Bring all to boil together.

*Dosage:*    ½ a glass twice daily.

## 24. *Pneumonia*

Pneumonia is an inflammation of the lungs, caused by an infection from bacteria or viruses. When one lung is affected, it is called Lobar pneumonia. When both lungs are affected, it is called bronchi pneumonia

### *Symptoms*

1. Sudden chills with violent shivering.
2. Blood stained sputum
3. High fever
4. Palpitation
5. Burning sensation on one or both sides of the chest. At times it becomes difficult to lie down or sit for longs period of time because of the pain
6. Constant weakness and tiredness
7. Vomiting

### *Treatment*

## *Materials*

1.  Bitter leaf
2.  Honey
3.  Water

*Recipe:*    Simply squeeze some bitter leaf in water. Add 1 bottle of honey to 10 liters of the bitter leaf extract.

*Dosage:*    Take 1 glassful three times daily for 1 month

## *Formula II*
## *Materials:*

1.  6 pawpaw leaves.
2.  10 handfuls Lemon peels
3.  5 bulbs of garlic
4.  5 bulbs of onion
5.  10 liters of water:

*Recipe:*    Bring all to boil together.

*Dosage:*    Take1 glassful three times daily for 3 weeks.

## 25. *Tuberculosis*

T.B, as it is commonly called, is a communicable disease caused by Mycobacterium tuberculosis. The bacteria spread gradually in the body from the lungs to other organs such as the kidney, spinal cord, heart and bones.

## Symptoms

1. Fatigue tiredness
2. Loss of weight
3. Heavy sweating and perspiration at night
4. Coughing up blood-stained sputum

## Treatment

### Formula I
### Materials

1. *Gmelina arborea* (10 handfuls)
   Common name: Gmelina, Kashmir tree.
2. Pawpaw (10 handfuls)
3. Bitter leaf (10 handfuls)
4. 10 liters water

**Recipe:**   Bring all to boil

**Dosage:**   Take1 glassful three times daily for 6 months.

## 26. Hypertension

Blood pressure is the amount of pressure that is exerted on the arteries of the body as the blood circulates round the system. The human body is so constituted that, there must be a balance between the contraction of the left ventricle of the heart and the amount of blood pumped out into the aorta. When the pressure that the blood exerts on the blood vessels is consistently and abnormally high, it is called hypertension, when it is consistently and abnormally low, it is called hypotension. The human blood pressure varies during the course of the day. The blood pressure goes up during physical exercise, or while doing serious brainwork or if one is excessively worried. The blood pressure is at its lowest during sleep. The only reliable way to measure the blood pressure is by using the sphygmomanometer. The best time to measure blood pressure is in the morning, shortly after rising, A blood pressure of 135/70mmHg or 140/70mmHg is considered normal. A blood pressure of 140/90 is considered slightly high. A blood pressure of 150/90 or 150/100 is considered very severe and high.

## Causes

There are two types of hypertension. They are, Essential and Secondary hypertension. Essential hypertension is that which has no apparent cause, it just occurs. This is the case in 80-90% hypertension cases. Secondary hypertension is that which is caused by an underlying disease such as diabetes or kidney problems. The following are some of the probable causes of hypertension:

### 1. Heredity

Opinions differ on the role of heredity in hypertension. From clinical observations, however, there is enough reason to conclude that hypertension runs in families. For example, in a family where both parents suffer from hypertension, there is a 60-80 % possibility that one or two of their children will also develop the sickness. Some other opinions insist that what is inherited is the tendency towards the sickness, not the sickness itself.

## 2. Environment

We are products of our environments. Our dietary habits are conditioned by our social and cultural upbringing. Those who were brought up on high calorie diets are likely to develop hypertension. High intake of salt also leads to hypertension.

## 3. Mental Attitudes

Negative attitudes to life, hatred, envy, anxiety, excessive worry, are unhealthy mental attitudes. Persons in this state of mind are prone to getting severe hypertension.

## Treatment

### Formula I
### Materials

A. *Talinum triangulare*

English-Water leaf
Igbo-Ntu oka, ofe bekee
Yoruba-Gbure

B. 10 liters of water

**Recipe:**    Cut the roots into pieces. Measure 10 handfuls of the roots into B and bring to boil.

**Dosage:**    Take 1/2 a glass twice daily for two months

### Formula II

## *Materials*

    A. 10 bulbs of garlic
    B. 2 bottles of coconut water
    C. 4 bottles of water

**Recipe:**    Mix B and C together and blend with A.

**Dosage:**    1 shot three times daily for 4 weeks.

Another highly effective remedy for hypertension is *Ficus asperifolia*, called sandpaper tree in English, Asesa in Igbo, Epin in Yoruba, Baure in Esan. Squeeze the fresh leaves in water (like bitter leaf). Drink a glassful three times daily.

# CHAPTER NINE

# TRADITIONAL-MEDICAL GYNAECOLOGY

**PSALM 8**

*How great is your name, O Lord our God,*
*Through all the earth!*

*Your majesty is praised above the heavens;*
*Even when human beings claim that you are dead*
*The forests, the mountains, the hills*
*All radiate the splendor of your glory.*

*When I look at life*
*With all its mysteries and paradoxes,*
*I marvel at how little understanding human beings have*
*How limited is their knowledge!*

*Yet you have made them masters of their lives,*
*Gave them power to transform the earth*
*By faith not fear*
*By hope not despair*
*By love not hatred.*

*Life and death*
*Pain and suffering,*
*Joy and sorrow*
*All of these point to you*
*And are reconciled in you.*

*How great is your name, O Lord our God,*
*Through all the earth!*

## THE GLORY OF WOMANHOOD

In the book of Genesis, we have an account of the creation of the world. In the beginning, there was no Life. The earth was a formless void. Then God, in God's own free will, created the earth and everything in it. The accounts of creation in Genesis are fruits of years of reflection by Israelite writers on the wonder and mystery of the world. The world is so well ordered, everything fits so well together that one cannot but marvel at the wisdom of God.

The earth rotates round the sun in perfect equilibrium. If our earth had been a little bit closer to the sun it would have been too hot for habitation. If on the other hand the earth had been a little bit further away from the sun, it would have been too cold for habitation. Human beings and the plants exchange oxygen and carbon dioxide in such a balanced way that life continues. In this system, there is no inferior or superior. We exist together.

We exist together, human beings, plants, animals and spirits are harmonious vibrations of the music called life. Day and night follow each other. The seasons come and go, the plants and animals are so varied, yet each species is unique and beautiful. The rivers flow. The wind blows. The sky shows forth its beauty. The forests tremble. The universe is beautiful in a complex way. Having created heaven and earth, and the other creatures, God now created man and woman. The human species thus became the youngest entity in the universe. God created the human species as a reflection and summary of the complex nature of the cosmos. Human beings are the perfect conclusion of creation.

The human body reflects the complexity and mystery of the universe. There is no other entity as perfectly modeled as the human body. When we look at the universe, we notice a certain rhythm, the rhythm of night and day, rainfall and sunshine, winter and summer, cold and heat, and finally planting and harvesting. If this rhythm is disturbed, there will be chaos, disharmony and disease. The same rhythm that sustains the universe also governs the human body. This is especially true of the female body. The female body is as complex, mysterious and marvelous as the cosmos itself. The secret of the allurement and magnetism of women lies in their closeness to nature. The further women drift away from nature, the weaker they become.

Women radiate such powerful magnetism that men and even animals are attracted to them. Women are so subtle and sensitive that they can easily perceive people's feelings more than men do. While men are more attracted by sight, the sight of a beautiful face or figure; women are more attracted by other inner and deeper qualities like the tone or quality of a man's voice, or his bodily gestures. A gentle touch, an honest expression, an appreciative look, attracts a woman more than mere physical appearance. Most often, when men tell lies, women find it easy to detect because of their sensitive nature. What a special privilege it is to be a woman! The glory of God and creation is a woman fully in touch with herself and with nature. So often you see some women struggling with men, as if men are superior human species who pass some attributes which women are deprived of. What a pity! Know yourself. Be at one with yourself. Allow your body to follow its own natural rhythm, and then you will discover how powerful you are.

When you wake up in the morning, drink three or four cups of water. For breakfast, take only raw fruit. Only drink water an hour before or after meals. Do not drink while eating. If you find this difficult, then take as little as possible. Endeavour to drink at least four liters of water daily. Your monthly menstrual circle is not a curse. It is God's wonderful work.

Even as the universe has its seasons, each one following the other, so also does your body. Follow this rhythm Woman, and it shall be well with you. Do not tamper with it. Your diet, your lifestyle, your thought pattern must contribute to the proper functioning of your body. Avoid overcooked food. The more natural your diet, the better for you.

Junk foods such as, biscuits, ice creams, sugar, chocolate and coffee disrupt the proper functioning of your system. Try as much as possible to avoid them. Eat fruits such as, pawpaw, plantain, banana, and many others. Eat plenty of vegetables. When you eat rice, beans or yam, eat them with vegetables. It often happens that some women experience pain during their monthly menses. In fact, majority of women experience different degrees of pain before, during or after menstruation. At times, the pain can be very severe, so severe that they curse themselves for being women. Your pains are not your pains. They are life expressing life in you. Your pain is life longing to multiply itself saying, 'I am one, let me be many'. Women who suffer from painful menstruation should collect the fresh bark of the plant, *Alstonia boonei*, which Igbos call Egbu, Yorubas call Ahun, Binis call Ukhu, Esan people call Ojegbukhun, Urhobos call Ukpukuhu, and Efiks call Ukpo. Fill a medium-sized pot with the bark and then fill with water. Bring to boil. Allow it to stand for 24 hours, then sieve. Add 1 liter of honey to 4 liters of the preparation or 2 liters of honey to 8 liters of the preparation, and vice versa.

The dosage is half a glass three times daily. Begin medication one week before your menstruation. Continue until the menstruation is over. Do not expect a complete disappearance of pain the first time of using this medication. You will experience a gradual disappearance of pain each month. Nowadays, one hears a lot of women complain of irregularity of menstruation, scanty menstrual flows, miscarriage, lack of menstruation (Amenorrhea) and discoloration of menstrual blood (the color changes from red to dark brown). If you suffer from any of the above named ailments or other related problems, you should get yourself familiar with the plant, *Newbouldia laevis*. Igbos calls it Ogirisi/ Ogrishi. Yorubas call it Akoko. Esan people call it Ukhimi. The Hausas call it Aduruku. Urhobos call it Ogiriki. The Efiks call it Obot. This plant, whose common name is fertility plant, is regarded in most places as a sacred plant. The Yorubas regard it as a royal plant, hence the leaves are often used in the blessing and coronation of a new chief or king. It is forbidden to use this tree for firewood. The leaves are evergreen. Every woman should become familiar with this wonderful plant. For varieties of gynecological problems, squeeze the leaves of *Newbouldia* in water (same way as bitter leaf). Take a glassful two times daily. This preparation is good for such ailments as irregular menstruation, miscarriage, scanty menstrual flow, painful menstruation, (Dysmenorrhea), suppression of menses (Amenorrhea) and discoloration of menses. If you suffer from excessive menstrual flow, or short menstrual interval, collect the bark of the fertility plant, put it in a medium-sized pot and then fill the pot with water and bring to boil. Then allow it to stand for 12 hours, then sieve. Dosage is half a glass two times daily for 6 weeks. The earth is a mother, exceedingly fertile. Women are co-creators with God. They radiate the beauty and complexity of the cosmos. Women are mothers of the cosmos. May women discover their dignity, so that the world may be a better place.

## THE PROBLEM OF INFERTILITY

Patricia is a young lady of twenty-nine. She and her husband have been married for five years but have no children. Patricia works in a big company, while her husband is a successful bank manager. Joseph and Patricia were not anxious to have a baby in the first year of their marriage, since they wanted to settle down fully. However, when the first year ran into the second and still no pregnancy, they became agitated. Their parents began to raise eyebrows. By the third year of their marriage anxiety had taken over the honeymoon bliss. Patricia began to pay a series of visits to different hospitals. She had all sorts of laboratory tests and physical examinations. After each test, Patricia was always told that she had no problem and yet was always given dozens of tablets and capsules to swallow, by the fourth year of their marriage, Joseph, Patricia's husband was asked to go for medical examination. He bluntly refused, saying that he had no problem. He argued that if his wife were treated with more drugs, nothing would stop them from having a child. Both Joseph and his parents continued to point fingers at Patricia, saying she was barren. They even threatened to marry a new wife for Joseph, if Patricia does not conceive soon. This was the state of things when he met Patricia. A once cheerful and happy-looking lady, had fallen into depression. She is just one among thousands of infertility cases in our society today. The issue of childless couples poses a big challenge to the Churches in Africa. How do we introduce the childless couples into the Church? How do we preach the Gospel to them? The task before African scholars and theologians is to evolve a theology that will help the childless couple to accept the reality of life with eschatological hope. In the Catholic tradition, marriage is first of all a bond of friendship between two people, that is man and woman. If this bond of friendship is blessed with the fruit of the womb, then the couples are to bring up their children in the fear of God. However, procreation should not be made the primary aim of marriage. Sadly, many African Christians do not agree with this teaching. For them, the primary aim of marriage is to have children. Marriage without children is no marriage. Within the Church, childless couples are made to feel abnormal and unaccepted.

Even the language we use and the societies we form in the Church make childless couples feel uncomfortable. We speak of Christian fathers and Christian mothers, reminding them that, until they have their own children, things are still not normal with for them.

## WHAT IS INFERTILITY?

A woman is said to be infertile when, for one reason or another, she is unable to conceive after a long period of trial. A man is said to be infertile when for one reason or another, he is unable to impregnate a woman.

## TYPES OF INFERTILITY

There are two types of infertility. The first type is called primary infertility. This refers to the inability of a woman to conceive at all, or of a man to impregnate a woman. The second type is called secondary infertility. This implies that there was a time when the man or woman was fertile but is no longer fertile. A woman may give birth to one or two children and suddenly find herself unable to be pregnant again. This is secondary infertility. Traditional gynecology is a specialist area that should not be delved into without proper training. Medical doctors trained in the western tradition should join hands with traditional healers to find solutions to infertility problems of our people. Precise diagnosis is important in the area of gynecology. Modern laboratory technology has brought a lot of improvement to treat illnesses. Traditional healers should make use of it. Whenever there is any case of infertility, it is important to finds out which one of the couple has complications. This investigation may lead to one of the following case

A. *When one of the couple is not well*

The woman may be suffering from such illnesses as ovarian cysts or anovulation. The man may have a low sperm count. In this case, attention should be focused on the partner concerned. If there is true love and cooperation between them, this should not cause any problem. One should encourage the other and trust in God. Men often find it difficult to accept that something is wrong with them especially with reference to fertility. Therefore they blame their wives.

B. ***When both partners are not well***

In this case the woman may have ovarian cysts, while the man has low sperm count. This case is more complicated than the first and requires cooperation and understanding between the couple. In one out of five infertility cases the problem is with both individuals.

C. ***When no diagnosis can be made***

This can be very frustrating. Many Christians are quick to attribute this to witchcraft or evil spirits, since there is no medical reason why they cannot achieve pregnancy. Many go and visit native doctors who will consult oracles to find out the cause of their problem. Most often, they are told that a relative or friend is responsible for their woes. Do not be deceived. Remain steadfast in your Christian faith and trust that God does not abandon God's own people.

## *Causes of female infertility*

1. *Unhealthy life styles*

I strongly believe that one of the major causes of infertility is the unhealthy life style of the people of today. We have drifted away from nature and we are paying dearly for it. We need to reexamine ourselves very well and look at our way of life, our philosophy of life and our relationship with God, with others, with ourselves and with our environment. We exploit our body, as if we are free to treat our body as we like. We eat and drink whatever we like. Rather than eating simple and natural foods that will give nourishment and life to the body, we eat precisely those foods that harm our body.

2. *Endometriosis*

This is (at times) a painful condition in which cells from the uterine lining implant themselves outside the uterus where they bleed during menstruation, leading to ovarian cysts, scarring and adhesions.

3. *Anovulation*

This is when ovulation fails to occur or when it is not regular. This could be caused by administering the wrong medication, emotional imbalance or a polycystic ovarian disease called stein-leventhal syndrome.

4. *Hormonal Deficiencies*

Insufficient production of progesterone, known as short luteal phase, is a common example. This may permit conception but prevent proper implantation and nourishment of a fertilized egg.

5. *Infection*

This leads to scarring and adhesions of the uterus, ovaries or fallopian tubes.

6. *Cervical Infection/Blockage*

This occurs when polyps or very thick mucus block the cervix and make it impassable.

7. *Uterine tumors/mal positioning*

An example of uterine tumor is fibroids. Fibroids may not prevent conception, but often leads to miscarriage. Mal positioning of the uterus also leads to miscarriage.

8. *Contraceptive pills and abortion*

Often I hear infertile women complaining that before they got married they took in or got pregnant very easily, but immediately after their marriage they cannot. What these troubled women do not know is that the contraceptive pills they used in the past, is a factor in their present predicament. Experience has shown me that most infertile women have undergone an abortion at least twice, usually performed by incompetent 'doctor". It should be made known to all our young unmarried daughters that they must never tamper with their wombs. For their own sake and for the sake of the world, they must preserve their fecundity.

9. *Spiritual weakness*

We, the people of today, are indeed weak in spirit. Weighed down by materialism and greed, we have lost the spiritual insight needed to resist the temptations of this world. Weakness of the spirit manifests itself in bodily weakness and disease. Orthodox medicine is gradually coming to terms with this reality. Natural medicine takes a holistic approach to illness. That is why many people now prefer natural medicine to synthetic drugs. What we need today is self-knowledge, to know ourselves as we are, so that we can really know God.

## Causes of male infertility

Apart from wrong life styles, spiritual weakness and other related factors, the following physical defects cause male infertility.

1. *Azoospermia*

This is an absence of living sperm in the body

2. *Oligospermia*

This is also called low sperm count or inadequate sperm. Related to this are other factors like motility (sperm swimming ability) and morphology (structure of the sperm cells).

3. *Infection*

This leads to sperm blockage. A lot of men suffer from one infection or another. The most common of infections are syphilis, staphylococcus and gonorrhea. If these infections are not well treated, they become resistant.

4. *Varicocele*

This occurs when varicose veins are grouped together in the scrotum.

5. *Undescended testicle*

This renders the testicle incapable of functioning. Serious accidents affecting the reproduction organs can also lead to infertility.

6. *Heat*

Working around hot ovens, wearing tight shorts or underwear, driving for very long hours can generate too much heat that may interfere with maturation of sperm.

## *Diagnostic tests*

Traditional medicine is highly effective in treating the sicknesses mentioned above. It is time for doctors trained in the Western system of healing to recognize and accept the fact that there are other equally effective methods of healing. Orthodox doctors need to be more humble and open-minded, so that they can work creatively with traditional healers. After all, most of our people now prefer traditional medicine to synthetic drugs. Moreover many of today's African orthodox doctors were brought up on traditional medicine, which is part of our heritage. To ignore this rich heritage would be a great tragedy. On the other hand, traditional healers should not claim that they can cure every illness.

Orthodox drugs are often very effective in acute illnesses that can kill in a short period of time. Traditional medicine is very effective in treating chronic illnesses, like diabetes, asthma, cancer, fertility problems and many others. The reason why traditional medicine failed in some areas is not because of a lack of useful herbs, but because of incorrect diagnosis. For example, whenever a man complains that he is infertile, many traditional healers do not bother to find out precisely what is wrong. In many cases they simply administer herbal remedies for impotence. But impotence does not make a man infertile. It only means that he has difficulty with penile erection. If the man's real problem is low sperm count, then the impotence medicine will not solve his problem. The following diagnostic tests will help to know exactly what the problem is For the man, the most common tests are; semen analysis, testicular biopsy and VDM to check for infection.

Most often the test recommended for the woman is the pelvic scan, to determine if the ovaries are of normal configuration and if there are uterine tumors. Besides the pelvic scan, perhaps the most common test for women is the keeping of a basal temperature chart. This involves making a daily record of one's temperature immediately upon walking. Ovulation is preceded by a slight rise in temperature. Keeping track of temperature fluctuations helps determine if and when ovulation is occurring. A woman may also be required to undergo hormonal analysis to determine the hormonal levels. Other tests include:

A. **Hysterosalpingogram**

This is done to check if the tubes are free and normal. Dye is injected through the cervix into the uterus and movement is monitored by X-ray. It is often very painful

B. **Hysteroscopy**

A procedure in which the cervix is dilated and the uterus distended to determine whether there are any intrauterine abnormalities.

C. **Laparoscopy**

A minor surgical procedure involving the insertion of a lighted telescopic instrument through a small incision just below the navel, giving the doctor a clear view of all pelvic organs.

D. **Culdoscopy**

This involves making an incision in the vaginal wall through which a telescopic tube is inserted to view the internal organs.

### *Natural remedies for infertility*

The principles are:

1. The more water you drink, the better for you.
2. The more fruits and vegetables you eat, the better for you.
3. The more natural your diet is, the better for you.

Learn to drink at least four glasses of water first thing in the morning daily. This is extremely important for infertile couples. If you cannot have your supper or dinner before 7.00 p.m. simply forget about it; and take plenty of water. Make sure you take no less than five cups of water daily. Men who suffer from low sperm count should avoid alcohol and sugar. They should take plenty of lime, lemon and honey. Women should avoid sugar and all sugar products like ice cream, minerals or soft drinks, or glucose.

Remember that a ball of orange is better than a bottle of coca-cola drink.

## 1. *Uterine hemorrhage*

### *Materials:*

   A.  10 half-ripe mango fruits
   B.  5 bottles of water
   C.  1 bottle of honey

   *Recipe:*    Peel the mango like an orange, grind the peel with water, then add the honey.

   *Dosage:*    Take1 shot twice daily for 1 month. Side effect: None

## 2. *Anovulation*

## *Formula I*
## <u>*Materials:*</u>

1.  Bark and root of *Newbouldia laevis*.

    - English: Fertility plant
    - Yoruba: Akoko
    - Igbo: Ogirishi
    - Esan: Ukhimi

2. *Ginger*

    *Recipe:*    Scrape the bark of the root & stem. Dry and grind into powder. Pour 1 teaspoon of the powder into a teacup of hot water, and then add ½ a teaspoon of powdered ginger. Allow it to infuse for 10-15minutes.

    *Dosage:*    Take 2 cups daily for 6 weeks.

## *Formula II*

## *Materials:*

A.  40 leaves of fertility plant.
B.  20 pieces of *Xylopia aethiopica*

    - Yoruba; Erunje
    - Igbo; Uda
    - Hausa; Kimba
    - Esan; Usira

C. 40 leaves of *Alstonia boneei* (stool wood)

D. 10 bottles of water

E. 2 bottles of honey

**Recipe**:    Bring A,B, and C to boil together in D. Allow it to stand for 24 hours. Sieve and add E.

**Dosage:**    Drink 1 cup 3 times daily [cup:240ml].Side effect: Slight laxative

## 3. *Irregular/painful Menstruation:*

## **Materials:**

A. 5 bulbs of garlic

B. 5 fingers of ginger

C. 2 bulbs of onions

D. 10pieces of *Capsicum frutescens*

English-African red pepper

Igbo-Ose Oyibo

Yoruba-Ata eiye

Hausa-barkono

Benin-Isie

E. 1 bottle of honey

F. 1 bottle of water

**Recipe:**    Grind all together with E and F.

*Dosage:*    Take 2 dessertspoons 3 times daily

*Side effect:* Slight stomach pain for ulcer patients. Take plenty of water to neutralize the effect.

## 4. *Low Sperm count*

*Materials:*

A. 10 of kola pods
B. 5 raw eggs
C. 2 bottles of lime juice
D. 1 bottle of water
E. 1 bottle of honey

*Recipe:*    Cut A into pieces. Blend 7 handfuls of the pieces with B, C, D and E, Mix very well. Do not refrigerate.

*Dosage:*    Take 1 shot twice daily for 3 months. Make fresh preparation as needed.

## 5. *Ovarian cysts/adhesions*

*Materials:*

A. 50 leaves of *Vernonia amygdaIina* (Bitter leaf)
B. 50leaves of *Newbouldia laevis* (Fertility plant)
C. 50 leaves of *Gmelina arborea* (Kashmir tree)
D. 8 bottles of water E. 1 bottle of honey

**Recipe:**    Pound and squeeze A, B and C in the water. Sieve and add E. Do not refrigerate.

**Dosage:**    Take1 glass 3 times daily for 2 months.

## 6. *Fibroid*

## *Materials:*

A.  30 pieces of fresh immature palm nuts
B.  30 pieces of *Spondias mombin*

    English-Hog plum
    Igbo-ljikara
    Yoruba-Akika, Iyeye
    Hausa-Tsadar masar
    Bini-Okhighan

C.  10 liters of water
D.  1 bottle of honey.

**Recipe:**    Bring A and B to boil. Allow it to stand for 12 hours. Sieve and add D.

**Dosage:**    Take 1/2 a glass 3 times daily for 4 months.

**Note:** *Do not take for more than 4 months.*

# THE PAINS OF IMPOTENCE

The medical Dictionary (Churchill Livingstone) defined impotence as an inability to participate in sexual intercourse. It can be due to lack of erection or premature ejaculation. Sexuality is an integral part of every human life. And when we speak about sexuality, we are not merely speaking about the act of sexual intercourse or coitus. Sexuality embraces every aspect of human life. Sexuality means relationship. We become persons by relating with others and we define ourselves only by relating with others. We all want to succeed in life, to be famous, to be strong. We all want to attain what we want to become what we want. We all have a great urge to do great things and to be successful. It is this desire that propels men and women to work and assert themselves, and without this urge, life would be lifeless, dull and boring. In the animal world, we notice a great desire for self-identity. Each animal knows its place and wishes to remain what it is. Each animal species has its own defense mechanism and survival instincts. Vitality is a characteristic of the animal kingdom. In the plant world, we notice a similar vitality and self determination. The force behind all these phenomena is the sexual energy. Sexual energy is what makes a man to set an ideal for himself and pursue it with vigor. This is what makes a man to endure intense hardship for the sake of a greater benefit. It is what draws a man and a woman together. It is what makes a particular type of music to appeal to this or that person. It is what propels living beings to hold on to life. It is the same energy that makes a monk to renounce the world so as to lose himself in unceasing contemplation of God.

The sexual energy is so tremendous that it needs to be controlled and channeled towards something good. Marriage is one of the most effective tools for controlling sexual energy. A man should love a woman by creatively loving and caring for his wife. Who also returns love for love. They both express their love and unity through, among others, sexual intercourse. A young unmarried man or woman is in constant danger of losing control over his/ her sexual urge. Coitus, that is, sexual intercourse, is one of the most effective ways of communicating love between married couples. When the sexual act is done outside wedlock, it leads to disharmony and distress. Sex is a language. It is an expression of complete trust, love and acceptance of the other. Many men understand sex to mean coitus that is, insertion of the penis into the vagina. What a wrong idea! Most women, on the other hand, see deeper than that. For a woman, touching, kissing, and other forms of fore play go into the definition of sex. Many men tend to see sex as penile insertion and ejaculation. This misconception has ruined so many families. The following are some of the many causes of impotence:

1. *Psychological*: Most often, impotence is caused by the state of mind of the sufferer. Such states as depression, anxiety and poor self image as well as lack of trust can lead to impotence.

2. *Physical Illness*: Impotence can result as a consequence of certain illnesses. One of such is Diabetes. Indeed, most diabetics have problem with penile erection. In such case, one should treat the cause rather than the effect. Fever, pile and venereal diseases can also lead to impotence.

3. ***Culture:*** Impotence tends to be common in some areas more than in others. Social upbringing and mentality play a big role in impotence. Some people grew up with the idea that sex is dirty and sinful, even in marriage. They believe that sex is only for pro-creation and not for pleasure, even in marriage. Those brought up with this mentality will sooner or later fall prey to impotence.

4. ***Diet:*** Dietary habits play's a big role in one sexual prowess. Some food promotes sexual urge, while some weakens it. Fruits such as unripe plantain, ripe pawpaw, honey, garlic and onion enhances libido.

5. ***Wrong Medication***: Men who are hooked on self-medication as well as alcoholics are liable to suffer from impotence.

### *What to do*

Impotence is becoming alarmingly common in our society today. Many married men are depressed because they are no longer capable of penile erection. Some can maintain erection only for a short time. Psychologists and sociologists alike agree that sexual problems lie at the basis of most family problems. Whenever a couple begins to quarrel and suspect each other, be rest assured that something is wrong with their sexual life. Many marriages have broken up because of impotence. For a man, there is nothing as humiliating and depressing as impotence.

# HERBAL REMEDIES FOR IMPOTENCE

Men who suffer from impotence should go for medical tests to rule out pile, diabetes, fever or veneral diseases. Aloe Vera is one of the most effective remedies for impotence. Cut the root of this plant into pieces. Soak two handfuls of the cut roots in two bottles of gin for ten days. Dilute with two bottles of water. If you take this preparation in the morning, you will notice an improvement in your penile erection by evening of the same day. This is a sure testimony to the effectiveness of Aloe root for impotence.

## *THE ALOE VERA FORMULA*

### *Materials*

    A. Roots of *Aloe vera*
    B. 1 bottle of gin
    C. Two bottles of water

    ***Recipe:***    Cut the roots into pieces. Soak three handfuls of the roots in B for ten days after which you now add C.

    ***Dosage:***    1 shot two times daily.

### *Kola nut pod*

Another effective remedy for impotence is the kola nut pod. Cut the fresh kola nut pod into pieces. Soak three handfuls of the pieces in two bottles of gin for ten days. Dilute with one bottle of water and one bottle of honey. Take one shot four times daily.

## COPING WITH MENOPAUSE

### What is Menopause?

Menopause is the particular point in time when the last menstruation occurs. This is the correct medical meaning of menopause. It refers to that specific point of cessation of menstruation. But in ordinary language, menopause embraces both the times before and after the exact time of menopause. In medical terms this is called Climacteric. In this work, we shall use the term menopause in the ordinary sense, that is covering the pre-and post-menstrual periods.

## SYMPTOMS OF MENOPAUSE

At puberty, the cells surrounding each egg in the ovaries form a follicle and produce two types of hormones, estrogen and progesterone. These hormones are vital to the reproductive life of a woman. It is these hormones that allow the eggs to be released. As from the age of 35, the production of estrogen begins to decline which means fewer eggs are released each month. From the ages of 44 and 48, menopause begins. Of course, this does not apply to everybody. Some women do not experience

menopause until they are in their fifties, while some experience menopause before the age of 44.

1. *Irregular menstruation:*

   The first symptom of menopause is change in the menstrual period. As from the age of 35 or 40, a woman may find that her period becomes irregular, or scanty," The flow may be excessive or prolonged. The period may come bi-monthly rather than month, or it may come every two weeks. All of these are signals to remind women that they cannot be fertile forever, that they are nearing menopause even though the actual menopause may be 10 or 12years away.

2. *Hot flashes*

   You are sleeping peacefully in your bed. Suddenly you wake up. Your body feels so hot that you think it is on fire. You begin to sweat profusely as if you have been running. You feel like stripping yourself naked or lock up yourself in a freezer. When you lie in your bed, the sheets are soaked with sweat. If you experience all or some of these symptoms, you are at menopause. These experiences can be disturbing to many women. Hot flashes at night result in insomnia. Women need to understand these symptoms so as to adapt properly to them.

3. *Aches and Pains:*

   Other symptoms of menopause are pains and aches all over the body. Some women have aches and pains before, but at menopause the pains increase. This is because of the decreased estrogen. Estrogen is the hormone that nourishes and strengthens the body tissues. Especially in the female genital track and the breasts. With the decline in Estrogen, the tissues become weaker and prone to infections. They become stiffer and aches and pains arise.

### 4. *Sensations*

It often happens that at menopause, a woman begins to experience some sensations all over the body. Some feel as if ants are crawling all over their body. Some feel sweats trickling down from their head to their cheeks, but often they reach to wipe it off, they feel nothing. Some feel tingling sensations in the face, and prickles and tingles running around the body. The decreasing estrogen causes all these. If you are a health worker, you will notice that all or most of the women who complain of these sensations are between the ages of 40 and 50.

### 5. *Vaginal dryness*

One effect of estrogen shortage is that the vaginal walls become dry and stiff. The walls become thin and lubrication diminishes or disappears altogether. The skin around the vulva becomes thin and dry and easily irritated. As time goes on, the vagina becomes shorter and narrower like that of a little girl. Sexual intercourse becomes very painful if not impossible.

## *Psychological effects of menopause*

We are not just bodies. We are also spirits. The proper description of the human person is an embodied spirit. Just as what goes on in our minds can affect our bodies, so also can what goes on inside our bodies affect our minds. This is especially true of women. For many women, menopause is accompanied by a sudden change in temperament. They become irritable and hot-tempered. They feel that their husbands no longer have interest in them like before. They feel that they are no longer as attractive as before. It is very important for men to understand their wives as they pass through this stage. Often, men do not understand what their wives are going through. This creates a lot of tension and division in families.

Secondly, menopausal women often experience depression, anxiety, and nervousness. This could be caused by a consciousness that they are aging. Some scientists have proposed that estrogen nurture both the mind and body. Hence, a decline in estrogen may result in depression, forgetfulness and nervousness. Whatever may be the cause, it is important to assure menopausal women that there is hope.

### Herbal aids for menopause

I wish to say emphatically at this juncture that menopause is not a disease. Menopause is only a stage in the life cycle of a woman. To many women who are going through menopause, I want to offer words of consolation and encouragement. Your body is beautiful. Everything, every creature is beautiful. Menopause can be liberating experience, and I know of many menopausal women who are happy and are enjoying it. What you need is an understanding of yourself and a stronger faith in God.

The secret of living an enjoyable and meaningful life after menopause is to take care of the body early in life. We often are like a man who said on his seventieth birthday, "If I knew I would live so long, I would have taken better care of my body". We should take care of our body early in life so that it can serve us better at old age. The importance of water for proper functioning of the body cannot be over emphasized. Early in the morning, on rising from bed, drink three to four cups of water. It is not enough to do this for a month or two. Make it a habit. If you are able to do this continually for a year, you will see what a transformation will come upon your body. Let our young women keep this in mind rather than wait until old age sets in.

As for those nearing menopause, we also affirm that water is a great help. Take as described above. You will soon notice a reduction in hot flashes and internal heat. Bitter leaf is one of the best women friendly plants around. Anywhere I go I never fail to emphasize the importance of bitter leaf plant for health. Bitter leaf is excellent for the body either before, during or after menopause. Bitter leaf takes care of such symptoms as hot flashes, internal heat and rheumatism. With bitter leaf around, women do not need to take artificial estrogen, which in any case has its own negative side effects.

The body can take care of itself if only we allow it. Bitter leaf does not supply estrogen but helps the body to produce the amount of estrogen needed for life. Squeeze the fresh leaves in water. Take a glass every morning and night. This is good for those who are already experiencing symptoms of menopause as well as those who have attained menopause.

Younger women in their mid-thirties should take a glass of bitter leaf extract every night. Make it a habit. It is however important for those who take bitter leaf extract to check their urine and blood sugar level from time to time, since the bitter leaf solution can lower urine and blood sugar levels. Menopausal women should take plenty of honey. A lot has been said and written about honey. Those who take honey regularly will remain fresh and healthy and strong till old age. They will go through menopause without falling victims of the symptoms. Mix four dessert spoons of honey with 1/2 glass of water and drink twice daily.

Another useful herbal preparation to ease the symptoms of menopause is the wonder tincture. It is call wonder tincture because of its effectiveness.

### How to prepare wonder tincture

### Materials

    A. 5 bulbs of garlic
    B. 5 pieces of ginger
    C. 2 liters of dry gin

**Recipe:** Cut A & B into tiny pieces and soak in C for two weeks. Keep container tightly sealed.

**Dosage:** Two dessertspoons every night.

# CHAPTER TEN
# HERBS AND THEIR USES

1. *Alliums cape*

English—Onion, Igbo-Abase, Yoruba-Alamosa, Hausa

*Parts used:* Leaves, bulb.

Contains: Riboflavin.

*Medicinal Values:*

1. *Insomnia:* Chew 1 bulb every night.
2. *Loss Of Memory:* Chew ½ a bulb every morning and night
3. *Hypertension:* Grind/blend 5 bulbs of onions with 1 bottle of honey. Take 4 dessertspoons twice daily.
4. *Diabetes:* Chew 1 bulb every morning and night.
5. *Headache:* Crush 1 bulb and press out the juice. Rub on the forehead.
6. *Cough/Cold*: Mix juice with honey and take 2 dessert spoons twice daily.

2. *Alliums sativum*

English-Garlic,
Igbo-Ayo,
Yoruba-Aye,

Hausa-Tafamuwa

**Contains:** Saponins, Tannins.

**Medicinal Values:**

1.  **Asthma/cough/Worms**: Grind 5 bulbs with 1/2 bottle of honey. Take 2 dessert spoons thrice daily.
2.  **Epilepsy:** Chew 5 cloves of garlic every night.
3.  **Allergy/Arthritis:** For skin infections of all kinds, crush some garlic, press out the juice and apply to the affected parts. For Arthritis, apply the juice to the painful parts.
3.  **Ananas comosus**

English: Pineapple

**Contains:** Bromeline

**Medicinal Values**

1.  **Indigestion:** Drink 1/2 a glass of unripe pineapple juice every night, preferably on empty stomach.
2.  **Amenorrhea**: Boil 4 unripe pineapple fruits (peels inclusive) in 10 bottles of water. Drink 5 glasses daily.
3.  **Vitamin C Deficiency:** Drink a lot of ripe pineapple juice.
4.  **Skin Infections:** For eczema, black skin spots, etc, apply the pineapple juice to the affected parts of the skin.

## 4. *Alstonia boonei*

English-Stool wood,
Igbo-Egbu,
Yoruba-Ahun,
Esan-Ojegbokun

*Contains:* Alkaloids, echitamine, tannins, and saponin

## Medicinal Values

1. *Fever:* Fill a small pot with the bark and bring to boil. Take a glass twice daily
2. *Diabetes:* Boil the fresh leaves and take a glass thrice daily for diabetes.
3. *Convulsion:* Soak the freshly cut bark in warm water for 12hours. Take a glass twice daily.
4. *Arthritis:* Boil roots and barks and allow to stand for24 hours. Take ½ a glass twice daily.

## 5. *Anacardium occidentale*

English-Cashew

*Contains:* Anacardic acid. Phenols, Tannins. Phenols.

## Medicinal Values:

1. *Malaria:* Boil the bark and take ½ a glass thrice daily: This is especially good for resistant malaria.

2. *Diabetes:* Cashew bark is scientifically confirmed to be very good for diabetes. Boil the bark and take a glass four times daily.

3. *Dysentery:* Boil bark and leaves together and take ½ a glass thrice daily.

6. *Senna alata*

English-Ringworm plant.
Igbo-Okpo.
Yoruba-Asunwon.
Esan-Ojegbukhun:

*Contains:* Saponin, Tannins, and Azulene

*Medicinal Values:*

1. *Constipation:* Squeeze the tender leaves in water and take a glass every night for 4 days

2. *Skin Infections:* Mix the dried, powdered leaves with palm-kernel oil, and apply to the body for eczema, rashes and other skin ailments.

3. *Asthma/Bronchitis:* Boil the fresh leaves in water and take a ½ glass twice daily.

4. *Gonorrhea:* Boil the root with some garlic and onion. Take a ½ glass twice daily.

NB. Do not take this herb for more than a month.

## 7. *Citrus aurantifolia*

English-Lime,
Igbo-Afofanta,
Yoruba.-Osan-wewe,
Hausa-Lemu
***Contains:*** Essential Oil

### *Medicinal Values:*

***Fever:*** Bring the fresh leaves to boil and take a glass twice daily. For quicker result, mix with mango, cashew and need leaves.

***Jaundice:*** Boil the leaves with some pawpaw leaves. Take a 1/2 glass twice daily

***Typhoid:*** Boil the fruit rind and take a 1/2 glass thrice daily

***Headache:*** Pound the fresh leaves and press out the juice. Mix the pure, undiluted juices with onion juice and rub on the forehead. The headache disappears within a few minutes.

## 8. *Citrus limon*

English-Lemon;
Igbo-Oroma-nkirisi
***Contains:*** Pectin, Essential oil, Vitamin B2 and C

*Medicinal Values*

1. *General Body Weakness:* Boil the fruit rind and take a ½ glass twice daily.
2. *Sore-Throat:* Mix the juice with warm Water and use to gargle twice daily.
3. *Bronchitis:* Boil the peels and tender leaves together. Take a ½ glass thrice daily.
4. *Earache:* Crush the fresh leaves and press out the juice. Apply 2 drops of the undiluted juice to the ear twice daily.

## 9. *Cocos nucifera*

English-Coconut,

Igbo-Ake bake, Ake oyibo,

Yoruba-Agbon,

Esan-Uvie

*Contains:* Protein, Minerals, Glycerioles of caprylic, Stearic and Oleic acids, etc

*Medicinal Values*

1. *Bronchitis:* Boil the roots and take a 1/2 glass twice daily.
2. *Liver/Kidney ailments:* Boil the root with some lemon leaves and roots of bitter-leaf plant. Take a glass twice daily.
3. *General Ill-Health:* Coco-nut water is an effective health tonic and cleanser. It is a good remedy for food poison.
4. *Cancer:* Mix a bottle of coconut water with a bottle of honey and take a shot twice daily.

5. **Poor Memory:** Eat the white pulp of the immature coconut to improve the memory.

## 10. *Cola acuminata (&Nitida)*

English-Kola,
Igbo-Oji,
Yoruba-Obi,
Hausa-Goro

**Contains:** Alkaloids

**Medicinal Values**

1. **Insomnia:** squeeze the leaves in water and take a glass every night.
2. **Impotence:** Boil the bark in water and take a glass every night.

**Kola**

3. **Tiredness:** Mix 1 teaspoonful of the powdered nut with a little honey. Take every night.

## 11. *Cymbogon citratus*

English-lemon grass,
Yoruba-Waapa

*Contains:* Essential oils (especially myreene and citral), saponins, tannins, alkaloid.

## Medicinal Values

1. *Fever:* Boil the fresh leaves together with mango and cashew      leaves. Drink a glass thrice daily for 7 days.
2. *Rheumatism:* For rheumatism, prepare as above.
3. *Nervous Disorder:* Boil both leaves and roots in water and allow to stand for 12 hours. Drink a ½ glass thrice daily.
4. *Insecticide:* To repel insects, burn some dried leaves on a small tire.

## 12. *Euphorbia hirta:*

English-Asthma weed,
Igbo-Odane inenemili,
Yoruba-Emi-ile. Egele
Hausa-Nonan kurchiya

*Contains:* Euphorbol hexacozonate, Cycloar-tenol, Ingeno-triacetate, tinyatoxin-tannins, etc.

## Medicinal Values

1. *Asthma:* Collect the fresh leaves and dry(never dry leaves directly under the sun) Add one teaspoonful of the dried, powdered leaves into a cup of boiling water. The dosage is one cup twice daily.

2. ***Cough/Bronchitis/Pneumonia:*** grind the fresh leaves to boil and take a ½ glass twice daily for cough, and 2 glasses thrice daily for bronchitis/pneumonia.

3. ***Dysentery:*** Boil the fresh, leaves in water and take a glass thrice daily for 5 days.

4. ***Constipation:*** Pound the fresh leaves and add a little water. Squeeze out the juice and take a shot every night for 3 days. (please do not exceed 3days).

13. ***Eucalyptus officinalis:***

English-Fever Tree, Eucalyptus

***Contains:***   Essential oils. resin, tannin, cineole

## *Medicinal Values*

1. ***Urinary Tract Infection/Bronchitis***: Bring the fresh leaves to boil. Take ½ glass thrice daily for 7 days. (Please do not go beyond the stipulated days).

2. ***Asthma:*** Add a teaspoonful of the dried powdered leaves into a glass of boiling water. Allow to steep for 15 minutes. Dosage is two glasses twice daily.

3. ***Typhoid Fever:*** Prepare as in no.1 above. Dosage is 1 glass thrice daily for 5 days.

4. ***Insecticide:*** Burn the dry leaves in a room to repel flies and mosquitoes.

14. *Ficus asperifolia*

English-Sand paper tree,
Igbo-Asesa
Yoruba-epin,
Esan-Ameme,
Hausa-Baure

*Contains:* Tannins

*Medicinal Values*

1.  *Hypertension:* Squeeze the fresh leaves in water (like bitter leaf). Drink a glassful thrice daily.
2.  *Gonorrhea/Enlarged Spleen:* Fill a medium-sized pot with the bark. Add water to full the pot. Bring to boil. The dosage is 1/2 a glass thrice daily for two weeks.
3.  *Urinary Tract Infection:* Boil the root in water and take ½ a glass twice daily.
4.  *Anti-Hypertension:* The dried powdered leaf is an excellent anti-hypertension drug. Add a teaspoonful to a glass of boiling water and take two cups daily.

*Warning:* pregnant women must not take this herb.

15. *Garcinia kola*

English-Bitter Kola,

Igbo-Adi,

Yoruba-Orogbo.

Bini-edun

*Contains:* Kolaviron, flavonoids-apigenin, saponins, tannins, and resin.

## *Medicinal Values*

1. *Jaundice/Hepatitis:* The seed is an ingredient in the preparation for Jaundice/Hepatitis. Crush 10 seeds and soak in one beer bottle of water. Dosage is 4 table spoonfuls thrice daily.
2. *Impotence:* Boil the root with some garlic and ginger and allow to stand for 12 hours. Dosage is 1/2 a glass thrice daily.
3. *Anti-Poison*: For snake bites, food poison or poison of any kind. Chew two bitter-kola seeds on an empty stomach every night.

## 16. *Jatropha curcas*

English-Pig nut,

Igbo-Olulu-idu,

Yoruba—Botuje, Lapalapa,

Esan-Ughongbon

*Contains:* Resin, Curcin, Saponins, Tannins, Inulin etc.

## *Medicinal Values*

1. *Fibroid:* Boil the leaves and roots together with onion, garlic and ginger. Dosage is ½ a glass thrice daily for three months

2. ***Epilepsy/Convulsion***: Boil the roots with Tobacco leaves and garlic. Dosage is ½ a glass thrice daily.

3. ***Wounds:*** Apply the fresh latex to fresh wounds to stop the bleeding.

## 17. *Lantana camara*

English-Wild sage,

Hausa-Kimbar,

Yoruba-Eleku, Ewon agogo

***Contains:*** Alkaloids. Essential oil

## *Medicinal Values*

1. ***Hypertension/Nervousness:*** Boil the fresh Leaves in water and, drink one glass twice daily. This has been proved to be very effective for these ailments.

2. ***Convulsion:*** Prepare as in no. 1 above. Dosage is 1/2 a glass thrice daily.

## 18. *Mangifera indica*

Common name-Mango

***Contains:*** Tannins, resins, glycoside, and flavonoids

Medicinal Values

1. ***Bronchitis:*** Bring some fresh leaves to boil. Drink a glass twice daily.

2. *Malaria Fever:* The fresh leaves boiled together with the leaves of Pawpaw, Neem (dogoyaro), Cashew and bitter leaf plant, is good for malaria fever.

3. *Anaemia:* Bring some quantity of the stem bark to boil. The dosage is ½ a glass twice daily.

4. *Diabetes:* Fill a medium sized pot with the fresh, tender leaves and bring to boil. Drink a glassful thrice daily.

## 19. *Momordica charantia*

English-African Cucumber,

Igbo-Alo ose,

Yoruba-Ejirin-wewe.

*Contains:*   Alkaloids, Mimordicine, Saponins, Charantin, Oleic acid.

### *Medicinal Values*

1. *Diabetes:* Squeeze the fresh leaves in water and drink one glass thrice daily. Many people have felt effectiveness of this preparation for diabetes.

2. *Constipation:* prepare as above and drink two glasses every night.

3. *Convulsion:* Make an infusion of the fresh leaves together with bitter leaves. Drink one glassful twice daily.

## 20. *Morinda lucida*

African Cucumber

English-Brimstone tree,

Igbo-Eze-ogu,

Yoruba-Oruwo,

Es-an-Ogo

*Contains:* Anthraquinones, Glycosides

Medicinal Values

1. *Diabetes:* Squeeze the fresh leaves in water together with bitter leaves. The dosage is one glassful thrice daily.
2. *Jaundice:* Fill a medium-sized pot with the roots and bring to boil with some pawpaw leaves and Lemon peels. Drink ½ a glass twice daily.
3. *Fever:* Boil the fresh stem bark in water and take one glassful twice daily.

21. *Musa paradisiaca*

English-Plantain,

Igbo-Ogadejioke, Ojioko,

Yoruba-Ogede agbagba,

Hausa-Ayaba,

Bini-Ogheda.

*Contains:* Inulin, Tanninsand Alkaloids

*Medicinal Values:*

1. *Kidney Infection:* Crush the root and squeeze out the juice. Drink four tablespoons thrice daily.

2. *Goitre*: For goiter, prepare as above. Mix ½ bottle of the pure juice with ½ bottle of honey. The dose is three tablespoonfuls thrice daily, increase the dose if required.

3. *Heart Problem:* Bring some amount of the fresh leaves to boil. Drink one glass twice daily.

4. *Intestinal Ulcer:* Dry the peel and grind into powder. Mix one table spoon of the powder with four tablespoons of honey, lick.

5. *Anaemia:* Boil some quantity of the root and drink ½ a glass twice daily.

## 22. *Nicotiana tabacum*

English-Tobacco,

Igbo-Otaba,

Yoruba-Ewe taba,

Hausa-Taba,

Bini-Itaba

*Contains:* Saponin, Tannins, Inulin, Nicotine Tobacco

## *Medicinal Values*

1. **Epilepsy:** Boil 10leaves and 10bulbs of garlic in 10 liters of water. The dose is ½ a glass twice daily.

2. *Depression:* Prepare as above. Drink ½ a glass every night.

3. *Anaemia:* Mix 6 tablespoons of dried powdered tobacco leaves with one bottle of honey. The dose is two tablespoons thrice daily.

23. *Psidium guasava*

Common name-Guava

*Contains:* Tannins, Resin, Essential oils,

*Medicinal Values:*

1. *Stomach Ache:* Chew some tender leaves. This brings a quick relief.
2. *Diarrhoea:* Bring some fresh leaves to boil. Drink ½ a glass twice daily.
3. *Irregular Menstruation:* Boil the stem bark together with some fresh ginger. Drink ½ a glass twice daily.

24. *Rauwolfia vomitoria*

English-Swizzlestick,

Igbo-Akanta,
Yoruba-Asofeyeje,
Es-an-Ukheta

*Contains:* Saponin, Rauwolfine, Reserpine, and Serposterol

*Medicinal Values:*

1. *Hypertension:* Scrape off the root-bark and allow to dry. Pour one teaspoonful of the powdered root into a glass of boiling water. Allow it to cool. The dose is two cups daily.

2. ***Impotence:*** Boil the fresh root in water. Drink ½ a glass every night.

3. ***Insomnia:*** Prepare as in no.1 above. Drink a glass every night. If case is serious drink two glasses, but never more than that.

4. ***Nervous Disorder:*** Prepare as in 1 above. The dose is one glass thrice daily.

## 25. *Sida acuta*

Igbo-Udo,
Yoruba-Iseketu

***Contains:*** Tannins, Saponins

## *Medicinal Values:*

1. Arthritis: Bring the fresh leaves to boil. Drink ½ a glass thrice daily.

2. Malaria Fever: Prepare as above. The dose is one glassful thrice daily.

3. General Weakness: Prepare as above. Dosage: One glassful thrice daily.

4. Kidney Problems: Fill a medium-sized pot with the root and water. Bring to boil. The dose is ½ a glass twice daily.

## 26. *Spondias mombin*

English-Hog Plum,
Igbo-Ijikara,

Yoruba-Akika, Iyeye,

Bini-Okhighan,

Hausa-Tsadar masar

*Contains:* Saponin, Tannins, Resin, Alkaloids

*Medicinal Values:*

1. *Fibroid:* Boil the seeds together with immature palm-nuts. Drink ½ a glass thrice daily
2. *Cataract:* Crush the fresh leaves and press out the juice. Add one teaspoonful of Lime juice to two tablespoonful of *Spondias* juice. Apply a drop to the eye twice daily.
3. *Gonorrhoea:* Bring the fresh leaves to boil and drink one glassful thrice daily.

## 27. *Terminalia catappa*

Common name-Umbrella tree, Indian almond

*Contains:* Tannins, Essential oils

*Umbrella tree*

*Medicinal Values*

1. *Insomnia:* Bring the fresh leaves to boil. Drink 2 glassfuls every night.
2. *Veneral Diseases:* Bring the fresh stem bark to boil. The 1dose is ½ a glass twice daily.

3. ***Health Tonic:*** Soak two handfuls of the stem-bark in two bottles of gin for 10 days. Drink two tablespoonful's thrice daily.

## 28. *Viscum album*

Common name-Mistletoe

***Contains:*** Alkaloids, Tannins.

### *Medicinal Values:*

Useful for all kinds of ailments such as epilepsy, cancer, diabetes, nervous breakdown. Hypertension, liver problems, hepatitis, and all sorts of gynecological complaints.

***How To Use:*** Soak 4 to 7 leaves in a cup of lukewarm water overnight. The following morning, add a cup of hot water to it.

***Dosage:*** 1 cup in the morning, 1 cup at night. You may increase the dosage if it is required.

## 29. *Zeamays*

Common name-Corn

*Medicinal Values*

1. *Diabetes:* Add one handful of the silk to a liter of boiling water. Allow it to cool. The dose is one glassful thrice daily.
2. *Hypertension:* Prepare as in no.1 above. The dose is the same.
3. *Kidney Infection, Obesity, Heart Problem, and Oedema:* Prepare as in no.1 above. The dose is the same.

30. *Zinginber officinale*

Common name-Ginger

*Contains:* Essential oil

*Medicinal Values:*

1. *Cough, Asthma, Colds:* Mix 5 tablespoonfuls of powdered ginger with ½ a bottle of honey. The dose is two tablespoons thrice daily.
2. *Suppressed Menstruation, Painful menstruation:* Add one teaspoonful of powdered ginger to a cup of boiling water. Drink a cup twice daily.
3. *Jaundice, Hepatitis:* Prepare as in no.1 above. The dose is three tablespoonfuls four times daily

# THE DANCE OF LIFE

I woke up at break of day
The sun was sun
The trees were trees
The bushes were bushes
The animals were animals
Then something stirred in my inside
And the sun was no longer sun
The trees were no longer trees
The bushes were no longer bushes
The animals were no longer animals
And I heard in my insides
The music of love
And the animals began to sing
And the plants began to dance
And the bushes began to sway
Then I stood, and in my front laid paradise
And I was no longer me
For I was lost in the dance of life

# THE RIVER OF LIFE: ECHOES OF HEALING

Before you is a river. The river flows from the place beyond the veil, from the place beyond the beyond. The river flows from the beyond and runs through the four corners of the earth. The river is the oldest entity on earth. The river knows the truth about the earth. The river, having seen the nakedness of the cosmos, knows the secrets of the cosmos. The river contains the seed from which life sprouts. The river contains all the elements of life. When the river coughs, they generate powerful waves, which vibrate round the cosmos. The river is as old as life itself. The river knows a lot. At the bottom of the river are remnants of lost civilisations. The river knows many civilisations. The heart of the universe is in the river. Though in one place, the river is everywhere. The river is a carrier of life. The river is in you and you are in the river. '-he river is in your veins. Like the river, you exist from the beginning of the world. Like the river, in you are contained the elements of life. The river has memories of time past, of events beyond the event, of secretes behind the secret. The river has memories of the beginning.

The river is the blood that flows through your veins. The river is the elements that make up 70% of your body. The river contains the hidden knowledge of the cosmos. The river knows the secret of the cosmos. You are the river. You know the secret of the cosmos in you is contained the hidden knowledge of the universe. The river knows the secret of fire; therefore it is more powerful than fire. The river knows the secret of the wind; therefore it is more powerful than the wind.

Because the river knows the secret of the cosmos, it has power over it, for to know is to have power. The one who knows the secret of your being is the one who truly has power over you. Everything has a hidden name. In this name lies the secret of everything. Discover the name of an object, and you gain power over it. To know the name of a person or a thing is to have power over them. In the name is contained the story, the history, of anything. The one who knows the name is the one who knows. To have knowledge means to know the name of things, for knowledge without name is incomplete. Only by knowing the name of a thing can one master it, for there is no mastery without a name. The one who does not know the name of things is ignorant, while thinking that they know.

To know the name implies that you know how to pronounce it, for the one who knows and does not know how to pronounce does not truly know. The one who knows the name of death has power over death. The one who knows the name of sickness has power over sickness. The one who knows the name of a charm has power over it. The one who knows the name of an enemy has power over them. The one who knows the name of spirits has power over spirits. The one who knows the name of fear overcomes fear. The one who knows the name of envy has power over envy.

The name of sickness is health; for health is a nonsense state that makes sense only within the context of illness. The name of fear is courage; for what is fear but the initial doubts of a great soul about to climb up the steep hill of self-discovery? The name of hatred is love; for you do not know what love is until hatred has slaughtered your ego in the altar of self-giving. The name of death is life; for death is not an end but the beginning of a journey to the place. where mystery becomes knowledge. And the only explanation of death resides in the master book of life.

From memories of past civilisations and kingdoms, the river knows that solidity is an illusion. The one who is ignorant mistakes solidity for real. The one who knows not is led astray by solid attractions: handsome houses, magnificent mansions, glittering vehicles, resplendent cloths and

marvelous tools. The river, having known many civilisations and knowing the hidden knowledge beyond the beyond, makes nonsense of solidity, for fluidity is the nature of the cosmos. Everything flows, moves. Nothing is static, despite the appearance to the contrary.

The river adapts to every shape and so takes the shape or form of whatever it enters into. The river does not expect the other to adapt to itself because the river knows the wisdom of life. It is I, not the other, who need$ to change, says the river. It is I, not the other, who is responsible for my actions, reactions, feelings and situations, says the river.

The river runs through every corner of the cosmos. The river owes no one an apology for being a river. The river is the element of dissolution. And the river owes no one an apology for that. The river owes no one an apology for what it is. The river knows that the secret of happiness is to be what one is and remain true to what one is. For the river, yesterday is today and today is tomorrow.

The river lives yesterday and tomorrow in the present, for the river knows the true meaning of time.

The river is everywhere. The river is the plant. The river is the sky. The river is the mountains, the hills and the valleys. The river knows that everything came from the same place, belong to the same maker, and would go back to the source. You are I and I am you. We belong together. Yet I am not you because I am a unique being. But the very element that makes me unique is what also makes you unique. The river is never lonely because the river is everywhere. The river lives in at-one-ness with everything. The river does not run after anything because the river knows that everything comes back. Nothing goes away permanently. Everything always comes back.

The greatest tragedy in the world is not the world wars, or the great earthquakes, or the great famines and plagues. The greatest tragedy is that men and women die without knowing who they are. The greatest tragedy is that men and women live an unexamined life. The greatest tragedy is that men and women die without making use of their innate talents. You see a mountain and you marvel at its height? You gaze at a flower and you admire its beauty?

Would that you could tremble at the awesomeness of your personality! Would that you could marvel at the magnificent of your own being, which has the allurement of a thousand roses! Would that you could open wide your hands and embrace the spirit of the cosmos, and respond to her rhythm, drawing you to the cosmic circle" where you vibrate to the primordial music and become one with the universe; then are you truly healed!

# SELECTED BIBLIOGRAPHY

Adodo, Anselm (1998), *Herbs for healing. Receiving God's healing through nature.* Ilorin: Decency Printers.

Akobundu, Okezie & Agyawa (1987), *A handbook of West African weeds.* Ibadan: IITA,

Arthur, Kleinman (1980) *Patients and Healers in the Context of Culture*: USA: University of California Press

Barcroft, Alasdair (1996), *Aloe Vera. Nature's legendary healer.* London: Souvenir press

Bek, Lilla and Pullar, Philippa (1986), *The Seven Levels of Healing.* London: Rider.

Bhanot, T.R. (1995), *Know about common diseases.* Delhi: Dreamland Publications.

Brennan, Barbara Ann (1988), *Hands of Light. A Guide to Healing Through the Human Energy Field.* USA: Bantam Books.

Brown, Deni (1995), *The royal horticultural society encyclopedia of Herbs & their uses.* London: Dorling Kindersley Limited.

Clements, Harry (1973), *Self-treatment for hernia.* Northamptonshire, UK: Thorsons Publishers,

Collins, Harry (2010) *Tacit and Explicit Knowledge*: USA: The University of Chicago Press.

Conrad, Peter, (2007) *The Medicalization of Society: On The Transformation of Human Conditions into Treatable Disorders*: USA: John Hopkins University Press.

Conway, Sally (1990), *Menopause: help and hope for this passage.* Michigan: Pyranee Books.

Eason, Cassandra (2001), *Chakra Power for healing & harmony.* England: Quantum

Emoto, Masaru (2001), *The Hidden Messages in Water.* New York: Atria Books.

Engel, Cindy (2002), *Wild Health. How animals Keep themselves well and what we can Learn from them* London: Weidenfeld & Nicolson

Evans, Mark (1990), A *guide to herbal remedies.* England: Wigmore Publications.

Falase, A.O (1987), An *introduction to clinical diagnosis in the tropics.* Ibadan: Spectrum books.

Ferder, Fran, & Heagle, John (1997), *Your sexual self. Path to authentic intimacy.* Indiana: Notre Dame Press.

Fulder, Stephen (1997), *The Garlic Book. Nature's powerful healer.* New York: Avery publishing group.

Gala, D.R & Dhiren & Sanjay (1996), *Diabetes, high blood pressure without any fear*. Mumbai: Navneet Publications.

Gill, L.S (1992), *Ethnomedical uses of plants in Nigeria.* Benin City: UNIBEN Press.

Good, Byron (1994) *Medicine, Rationality and experience: An Anthropological Perspective*: USA: Cambridge University Press

Gregory, Cajete (2000) *Native Science: Natural Law of Interdependence:* New Mexico: Clear Light Publications.

Harrison, E. Lawrence and Jerome, Kagan (2006) *Developing Cultures: Essays on Cultural Change*: USA: Rout ledge.

Harrison, E. Lawrence (1992) *Who Prosper: How Cultural Values Shape Economic and Political Success:* USA: Basic Books.

Grand, Amanda Le, & Wondergem, Peter (1990), *Herbal medicine and health promotion. A comparative study of herbal drugs in primary health care.* Amsterdam: Royal Tropical Institute.

Gursche, Siegfried (1993), *Healing with herbal juices.* Canada: Alive books.

Hawthorn, Geoffrey (1970) *The Sociology of fertility.* London: Macmillan Press.

Hay, Louise, (1969) *Heal your body. The mental causes for physical illness & the metaphysical way to overcome them.* London: Edem Grove

Hirt, Martin, and M'pia Bindanda (1995), *Natural medicine in the tropics.* Anamed

Hoffmann, David (1983), *The new holistic herbal.* Massachusetts: Element books.

Isibor, Kingsley (1993), *The medicinal uses of plants.* Osogbo: Igbalaye Press.

Jones-Llewellyn, Derek (1998), *Everywoman. A gynecological guide for life.* London: Safari books.

Khan, HazratInayat (1991), *The Mysticism of Sound and Music.* London: Shambhala Publications.

Krishnapada, Swami (1996), *Spiritual Warrior. Uncovering Truths In Psychic Phenomena.* USA: HariNama Press.

Larkin, Mary (2011) *Social Aspects of Health, Illness and Healthcare*: UK: The McGraw Hill Companies.

Livingstone, Julie (2012) *Improvising Medicine: An African Oncology Ward in an Emerging Cancer Epidemic*: USA: Duke University Press.

Lindernbaum, Shirley and Lock, Margaret (1993) *Knowledge, Power and Practice. The Anthropology of Medicine and everyday life:* USA: University of California Press

Livingstone, Churchill (1987), *Pocket medical dictionary.* New York: Livingstone.

Lynne, Mc Taggart (1996) *What Doctors Don't Tell You: Great Britain*: Clays Ltd, St Ives Plc.

Mallon, Brenda (2001), *Venus Dreaming.* Dublin: Colour books Ltd

McGarey, Gladys Taylor (1997), *The Physician Within You. Medicine For The Millennium.* Florida, USA: Health Communications

McLeod, June (2000), *Colors of the Soul. Transform Your Life Through Colour Therapy.* London: Judy Piatikus

Michael, Gelfand (1971) *Diet and Tradition in an African Culture*: Great Britain: Longman Group Limited.

Mitchell, Charlotte, (1991), *Plant medicine. A guide to home use.* London: Amberwood Publishing Ltd

Nnabuchi, Nwankwo, (1987),*The conscience of God.* Enugu: Life paths press.

Nwokeabia, U. Hilary (2009) *Why Industrial Revolution By-Passes Africa: Knowledge System Perspective:* London: Adonis and Abbey Publishers.

Okafor, C. Francis (2011) *Critical issues In Nigeria's Development: Environment, Economy and Social Justice:* Ibadan: Spectrum Books Limited.

Ojo, O.A. and Briggs, Enang Bassey (1982) *A textbook for midwives in the tropics.* Accra: Gibrine publishing company

Osula, Charles (1984),*Your personal medical and sexual problems. Know your health.* Benin City: Ilupeju Press.

Patton, Alell (1966), *Physicians, Colonial racism and Diaspora in West Africa.* Florida: University of Florida Press.

Schreiber, David Servan (2007), *Anti-Cancer: A New Way of Life*: England: Clays Ltd, St Ives

Simpson, George (1980), *Yoruba religion and medicine in Ibadan.* Ibadan: University press.

Sofowora, Abayomi (1979), *African medicinal plants. Proceedings of a conference.* Ile-Ife: University Press.

Sofowora, Abayomi (1982), *Medicinal plants and traditional medicine in Africa.* Ibadan: Spectrum books, 1982

Thesis, Barbara & Peter, (1993)*The family herbal.* Vermont: Healing Arts Press.

Thompson, Melvgn (1976), *Cancer and the God of Love.* Great Britain: SCM Press

Ugwu, Kevin, (1999), *The Sexual revolution. A twentieth century mistake.* Akure: Don Bosco printing press.

Varkey, C.P. (1993) Be *Human Be Holy.* Bombay: St. Paul's press.

Way, Bruce (2000), *Healing Energies. Understanding and Using Hands-on Healing.* Australia: Simon &Schuster

White, Ruth (2002*), Energy Healing for Beginners. A step-by-step guide to the basics of spiritual healing.* London: Piatkus.

Wolfgang, Wirth (1996), *Healing with Aloe.* Steyr: Wilhelm Emsthaler

# INDEX

# INDEX OF HERBS IN THE BOOK

Made in the USA
San Bernardino, CA
15 August 2018